War Yoga
Zurxāne

War Yoga
Zurxāne

Written by Tom Billinge

Published by Sanctus Arya Press

First edition, published December 2023 by Sanctus Arya Press.

This work is copyrighted © 2023 by Tom Billinge.

All rights reserved. No part of this book may be reproduced or used in any manner without prior written permission of the copyright owner, except for the use of brief quotations in a review. To request permission, contact the publisher.

Paperback: 979-8-9896441-0-0

Hardcover: 979-8-9896441-1-7

Library of Congress number pending.

Editing and layout by Benjamin Sieghart.

Cover art by Tom Billinge.

Inside illustrations by Tom Billinge, except those taken from the public domain.

More at:

waryoga.com

tombillinge.com

sanctusarya.com

"The day of battle's come: my noble lords,
Where are your iron-piercing spears, your swords?
Now is the time to show your bravery
And turn our vengeance into victory."
Šahnāme

Table of Contents

Disclaimer	10
Acknowledgements	12
Author's Note	16
Note on Pronunciation	17
Part I: Theory	**19**
Introduction	20
The Indo-Iranian Cosmos	29
The Celestial Mountain	36
The Old Gods	39
Zarathuštra	46
Zoroastrianism	57
Mithra	70
Mithra's Warband	92
Fire and Water	100
Yima and the Northern Homeland	118
The Manifold Soul	125
The Cosmic War	135
The Greater Holy War	142
The Final Battle	151
The Coming of Islam	155
Ṣufī Metaphysics	161

Wisdom of the Rising Light	168
Luminous Night of the Emerald Vision	177
The Four Bodies	187
The WarYogin	191
Rostam	195
Part II: Practice	**208**
Pahlavāni and Javānmardi	209
Zurxāne	221
Hierarchy	235
Entering the Go'd	241
Šeno	247
Narmeš and Xamgiri	253
Mil	265
Pā Zadan	272
Čarx	277
Kabbāde	282
Sang	287
Košti-ye Pahlavāni	291
Competition	296
Regimen	298
Afterword	302
Appendix I	304
Appendix II	306
Glossary	312

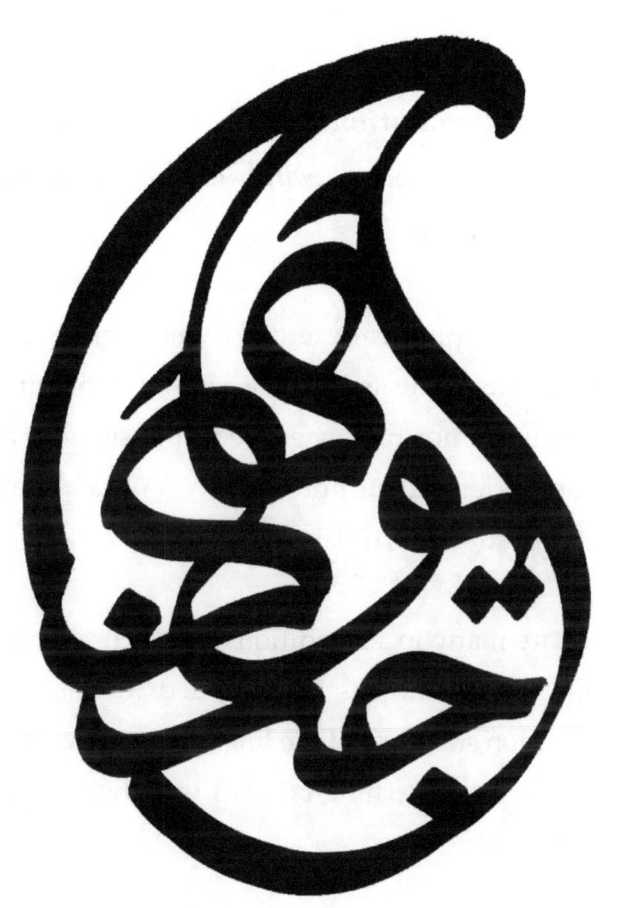

Disclaimer

"All these are illuminations which rise over the human soul when it is master of its body." Šehāb-al-dīn Yaḥyā Sohravardī, Book of Oriental Theosophy

WarYoga involves physical exercise, which carries inherent risk of injury. The contents of this work are for information purposes only, and neither the author nor publisher are responsible for any injuries sustained by the reader in their pursuit of WarYoga. All exercises are performed at the reader's own risk.

While there are many local traditions and techniques used in the *zurxāne* of Iran, the techniques propounded in this work are the accepted competition standard of the International Zurkhaneh Sports Federation. This is the governing body of worldwide *zurxāne* sports based in Tehran, Iran.

The names used for the exercises also have regional and local variations. However, the standard names used in Iranian competition have been utilised for this book.

For further information on the practices of WarYoga, visit **WarYoga.com**.

"Glory was created first and the body was created after. Glory was created in the body, fashioned for its proper function, and the body was created for its proper function." Bundahišn 14.8

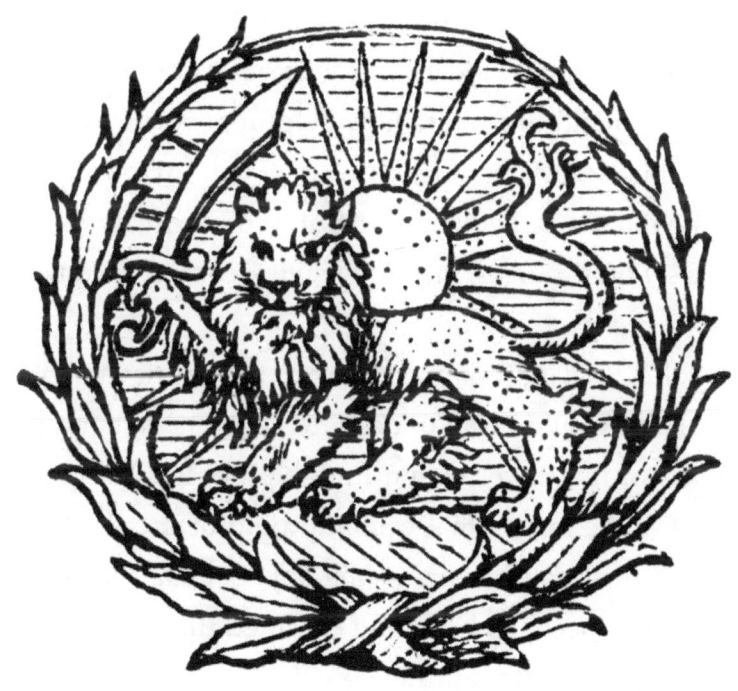

Acknowledgements

"Learn modesty, if you desire knowledge. A highland would never be irrigated by a river." Puryā-ye Vali, The Treasure of Truths

When I set out to research this book, I thought that a visit to Iran would be almost impossible given the state of international politics. It was due to a handful of incredibly helpful people that my difficult task became not only possible, but easy. First, my good friend and trailblazer who went before me, Paul Wolkowinski, gave me an invaluable set of resources, including a vital contact in Iran.

To say that Samane Tajalli was key to the journey to Iran and its various *zurxāne* would be an understatement. She not only arranged every aspect of my travel within Iran, but applied for my visa and dealt every single matter that came up both before and during my visit, even at unsociable hours of the day. Samane single-handedly took my specific needs in hand and executed them flawlessly. I owe her an immense debt of gratitude.

"Straightness is the means of acceptance with God. I saw no one lost on the straight road." Saʿdī Shīrāzī, Golestān

Accompanying me every step of the way as a guide, companion, translator, and friend was the indomitable Ariya Atashsoda. I met him as a stranger and left him as a family member. We shared much during my trip and Ariya made everything possible. He enabled me to gain deep insight from masters of *varzeš-e pahlavāni* – information that would have been impossible for me to access as a non-Farsi speaking foreigner. This book would be considerably poorer were it not for his diligence and understanding of what I needed.

While I visited many *zurxāne* in Iran, the first I went to invited me to enter the *go'd* and train with them. For this, I will always hold close to my heart Mr Hamid and all the *pahlavānān* at Zurxāne Šohadaye Farahazad in Tehran. Those great-hearted men welcomed me without reservation and made me feel one of them from the outset. I never felt out of place at any moment.

"Man, who is microcosm of the whole created universe, has the potential of total perfection." Šehāb-al-dīn Yaḥyā Sohravardī, The Shape of Light

My two incredible teachers at Zurxāne Mortazar Ali in Ardekan, Fars, gave me the gift of true *varzeš-e pahlavāni*. Both Azim Rahemi and Meysam Refahi are multiple time national champions in Iran. The profound depth of knowledge of those two men made the practice section of this book what it is. After many hours spent with both, I came to appreciate the beauty of the heroic sport more deeply than ever. Their love for *varzeš* is infectious and genuine. They live the ideals of *pahlavāni* and *javānmardi*.

Iran is a country that we in the West have been taught to look at through a lens of fear and suspicion. We have been told that its people are potential enemies. Having visited it and experienced firsthand what its people are like, I could not disagree with this sentiment more vehemently. The land is beautiful and welcoming. It is pure in a way that very few others are in this modern world.

The people of Iran are the kindest, most welcoming, most hospitable I have ever encountered in all my years of travel. They are painfully generous to the point that you become emotional and overwhelmed by their noble spirit. Though faced with various hardships, they do not allow these to change their fundamental character. They are too good, too kind, too genuine.

"Satan laughs at all your threats. What frightens him is to see a light in your heart." Ṣufī saying

In terms of resources, the online Encyclopaedia Iranica has been a critical resource. Built up over decades by eminent scholars, it is an unmatched resource for historical and other matters pertaining to Iran and Iranian culture. The body of work of prominent Iranologist Henry Corbin was indispensable to the sections on illuminationism and Iranian Ṣufī metaphysics.

Dr Manouchehr Moshtagh Khorasani was of great help in the very early planning stage for my first trip to Iran and his sublime book *Persian Archery and Swordsmanship* is an incredible work of scholarship. The translations from *The Scroll of Puryā-ye Vali* are his.

The image on the cover of this book is Persian calligraphy that reads "WarYoga." It is written in the design known in the West as paisley, but in Iran where it originates, it is called the *boteh*. The *boteh* represents the bent cypress tree and harkens back to the Zoroastrian tree of life, which makes one "he who always lives" – an immortal.

The cypress is a key emblem of the *zurxāne*. The cypress is strong, but bends; it resists but shows modesty. Because it is flexible as well as sturdy, it lives a long time. The heroes of the *zurxāne* aspire to the same principles: they aim for strength, morality, health, and modesty. The *boteh* is accordingly found on clothing and equipment associated with the *zurxāne*.

"Without wisdom, ability and rage together are like a sword eaten away by rust." Šahnāme

As always, I would like to thank my editor Benjamin Sieghart for his unflinching honesty and insight, and my wife Kristin for her unwavering support. Both of them are crucial to my work. I could not operate fully without either of them.

This book is dedicated to the *pahlavānān*, the holy warriors of Light and Truth.

Author's Note

"Men are enabled to improve and guide themselves in this world, to propagate with vigor their own race for the time of the final renovation." Dēnkard 3.209

As with the first WarYoga book, this is a work of two complementary parts. The first part is the theory section that lays out an historical, cultural, and mythological background. It is fertile metaphysical soil that is ready to receive the seed of the practical section that follows.

The philosophical and spiritual elements can be taken on without the physical action. Likewise, the exercises can be undertaken without the metaphysical structure. However, it is the union – the yoking of two halves – that makes for a powerful practice, joining mind and body as one and sending the Spirit to the eternal.

However you decide to use this book, I hope it is a positive force enabling you to move more powerfully through life.

"All this do we achieve; all this do we order; all these prayers do we utter, for the benefit of the bodies of mortals." Vīdēvdāt, 20.51

Notes on Pronunciation

"The home we seek is eternity; the Truth we seek is like the shoreless sea." Farīd ud-Dīn 'Aṭṭār, Conference of the Birds

Farsi, or Persian, is an Indo-European language, making it somewhat familiar to the ear of an English speaker. However, it still uses some more guttural sounds that are not utilised in English. Like modern English, it has also taken on loan words, particularly from Arabic.

This book has utilised the more modern transcription of Farsi and its ancient predecessors Avestan, and Old and Middle Persian. The non-Roman characters utilised by modern Avestan scholars have been avoided, as they would make the text much harder for the general reader to decipher. Some special characters have been used and are listed below, along with their pronunciation.

š - as in fi<u>sh</u>
č - as in <u>ch</u>eese
ā - as in f<u>a</u>ther
ē - as in d<u>ee</u>r
ī - as in f<u>ee</u>t
ō - as in b<u>oo</u>t

ū - as in m<u>u</u>te

x - as in lo<u>ch</u>: a throat rasp not used in English

ə - as in d<u>oe</u>s

Some specific examples are:

Xvarənah is pronounced "farr-uh-na" – the modern Persian word *"farr"* carries the same meaning

Činvatō Pərətu is pronounced "chin-va-too puh-ruh-tu"

Aša is pronounced "asha"

Zurxāne is pronounced "zur-ha-neh"

Šanāme is pronounced "sha-na-meh"

"Forget the reason if you search for the Eternal." Muḥammad Shirin Maghrebi Tabrizi, Divan-e Shams-e Maghrebi

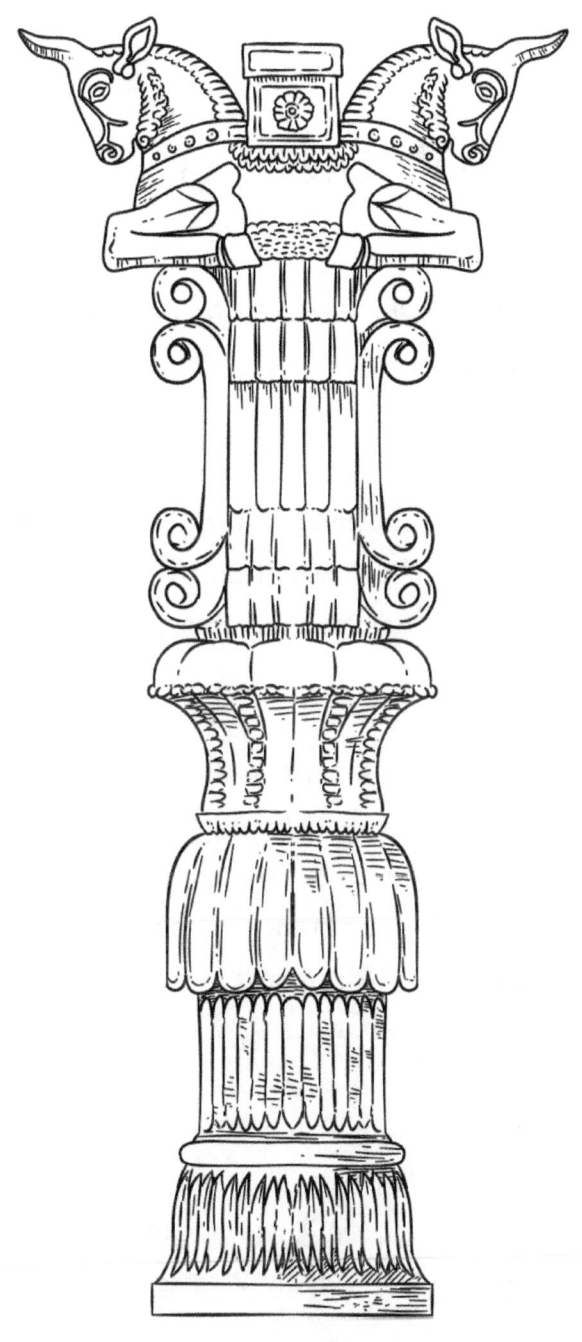

Part I: Theory

Introduction

"Hail to you, who are through your own power autonomous." Hōm Yašt, Yasna 10.25

The first WarYoga book explored the Vedic internalisation of the sacrifice. This second volume looks at the inner Cosmic War over the fruits of sacrifice through the lens of Iranian Tradition. Following the prescriptions of the initial volume, the WarYogin has already internalised the sacrifice.

He must now wage the inner Cosmic War against the forces of darkness to ensure his sacrificial offerings are accepted by the forces of Light. The internal sacrifice is expressed outwardly through the physical exercises of the Indic branch of the Indo-European martial metaphysical tradition. The inner Cosmic War is externalised through the Iranian heroic sport.

The outer war between Light and Darkness has been taking place since the end of the Golden Age. The war is becoming increasingly visible for those with eyes to see. This war cannot be won without the WarYogin fighting the Greater Holy War against dark forces found within.

While fighting his external foe, he must purge his being of the chaotic darkness casting a shadow on his brilliant inner divinity. Only once the WarYogin has purified himself of Ahrimanic elements within can he attain total internal and external victory.

"The turning of heavens have allowed me my life. My brother, you must know that our bodies are born to die and that warriors live to wear their helmets in war." Šahnāme

One of the great waves of Indo-European peoples that swept out of the original homeland were the Iranians, or as they still designate themselves today: the *Airya* ("Noble Ones"). While the term *Aryan* has fallen out of favour in the wake of the wars of the 20th century, it is a designation not only common to the various Iranian peoples, but to all Indo-Europeans as evidenced in the Indian *"ắrya"* and Greek *"aristoi."* In modern scholarship, *Aryan* is used in the term *Indo-Aryan*, referring to the Indo-European group that moved into northern India. This is distinct from the term *Indo-Iranian*, used to indicate the group that journeyed onto the Iranian plateau.

In the Iranian context the term *Airya* comes from the Proto-Indo-Iranian and Proto-Indo-Aryan **Áryas*, which in turn is derived from the Proto-Indo-European **heryós* ("member of our own group"). This is also the possible root of the word "hero" designating a guardian or protector. The country name Iran (Middle Persian *Ērān-vēj*) itself comes from the original Avestan *Airyanəm Vaējah* ("Expanse of the Airya"), which referred initially to the original homeland in the Far North.

As the new *Airyanəm Vaējah*, Iran was populated by a tapestry of *Aryan* people woven from centuries of invading northern nomadic tribes: the Proto-Iranian ancestors of the Medes, Sogdians, Persians, Parthians, Saka, and possibly the Hurrians, Kassites, and Mitanni. These Indo-European Steppe nomads moved in, raiding as the wolf cult warrior band, but eventually created their own kingdoms in this southern reflection of their original northern home. The mythos of all these people reflects a far northern point of origin that over time became too cold to inhabit, leading them to move south and west into India, Iran, and Europe.

"The demon of winter is more predominant in Eranvej. And it is declared by revelation, that in Eranvej there are ten months winter and two months summer, and even those two months of warm weather are cold as to water, cold as to earth, and cold as to plants." Dādestān-ī Mēnōg-ī Khrad 44.17-20

These groups became the new ruling elite, with their language and culture becoming dominant. These Indo-European people thrived on the harsh environment of the periphery – on the edge of survival. This tempered them so they flourished under hardship and pressure, distilling the holy warrior spirit. They brought with them mastery of the horse and metallurgy, as well as a martial and patriarchal system of governance distinctly stratified into three castes who were above the indigenous underclass. Absolute authority rested in the leader or king, and until the overthrow of the Shah in the late 1970s, the king in the Iranian-Islamic system was the infallible "shadow of God on earth."

To talk only of Persia when referring to this land and its culture is to use too narrow a lens. The modern country of Iran encompasses a broad spectrum of different *Aryan* peoples from the Persians in the south and the Medes in the north, to the mobile Scythians and their Ossetian and Albanian descendants in the Caucasus. All these groups had a profound impact on Greater Iran and its culture. Thus, to talk of a single Persian culture is a falsehood: the Iranian cultural sphere is a diverse and multifaceted gem.

"Unto ability is warriorship, that is, the most princely adornment of warriors is the ability which is expended, the manliness which is owing to self-possession." Škand Gumānīg Wizār 1.27

Iran has gone through many transitions, and changes in religion, but the original *Aryan* tradition has remained encoded in the spiritual forms that shaped themselves to the sensibilities of these people. A distinct vein runs through the religious expression of Iran and its people from the original Indo-Iranian religion through the Old Persian Religion, Zarathuštrian and Zoroastrian religions, all the way to modern Twelver Shī'a Islam. In fact, one could strongly argue that Iran was not subjugated to Islam, but that Islam conformed to the pre-existing Iranian cultural and spiritual tradition.

The heart feeding that vein lies deep in the Indo-Iranian past, possibly as ancient as the schism leading one major group into India and the other into Iran. This heart is the clear-cut differentiation between Light and Darkness, or good and evil. This found its clearest expression in the religion of the prophet Zarathuštra, to whom the *Gāthās* are attributed. The *Gāthās* are the oldest section of Zoroastrianism's holy scripture the *Avesta*. These *Gāthās*, along with the *Yasna Hapanghaīti* (another part of the *Avesta*) are written in Old Avestan – a language almost identical to Vedic Sanskrit, indicating an extremely ancient point of schism between Old Iranian and Vedic religions.

"Once those two Wills join battle, a man adopts life or non-life, the way of existence that will be his last: that of the wrongful the worst kind, but for the righteous one, best thought." Yasna 30.4

As this religion transformed into the somewhat syncretic Zoroastrianism, a duality endured. As Nestorian Christianity, Mahayana Buddhism, and Manichaeism all rose and fell in Iran, the battle between Light and Darkness remained at the centre of Iranian spiritual thought. When early Islam arrived, the Iranian scholars shaped the religion to their pre-existing traditions (while staying true to the *Qoran*), forming its intricate systems of laws and schools of thought into the religion known to the world today. It is not a coincidence that the esoteric Ṣufī tradition rooted in deeply to the fertile soil of the Iranian religious landscape.

It is out of this setting that the distinctly Iranian practice of *varzeš-e pahlavāni* or *varzeš-e bastani* and its associated *zurxāne* ("House of Strength") emerge as testing grounds for young holy warriors and as continued training for the mature warrior elite. This underground tradition emerged from the profound martial and spiritual experiences of Indo-European warriors. As discussed previously, the Proto-Indo-European word *heryós is the root of both *arya* and "hero." This finds its greatest expression in the *pahlavān* ("hero" or "champion"): the morally and physically superior athlete of the *zurxāne*. Just like his deepest ancestors, his title of hero is his sense both of his nobility and cultural identity.

"War, father of all things is also in us; he has hammered, chiselled, and hardened us to what we are. And always, as long as the spinning wheel of life continues to whirl within us, this war will be the axis." Ernst Jünger, War as an Inner Experience

The Iranian *zurxāne* – like the Indian *akhara* and the Greek *palaístra* – is a place where warriors, heroes, and athletes train. It is a sacred space that has had a home in the Indo-European warrior soul since time immortal. It is connected to the earth, with the original iterations of each being a simple patch of earth dug so men could wrestle for exercise, entertainment, prowess, settling disputes, and even as proxy warfare. This tradition comes down from the highest antiquity – from the Indo-Europeans themselves.

Over recent years, there has been a dispute between India and Iran as to who invented the exercises. Each lays claim to the origin. This is a false position on both sides of the argument.

The origin lies much deeper, from before either Iran or India existed. It was in a more primitive form, but the basic premises of the institutions and exercise methods came down from the shared *Aryan* ancestors of both modern Indians and Iranians. The reason that the

Indian and Iranian traditions share so much in common in terms of form is the cross-pollination that occurred over the millennia.

"To sleep is to remain satisfied with the false and ready-made opinions that everyone repeats. To wake (to be a 'Yaqzān' an Egregoros) is to become conscious of all the universe to which one can gain access only in a state of mystical waking (bīdārī)." Henry Corbin, Avicenna and the Visionary Recital

Geographically, the two modern countries, along with Afghanistan and Pakistan (both of which have an Indo-European heritage complete with the *akhara/zurxāne* tradition) have shared ever changing borders with each other. Iranian people (including the Saka Scythians, Alans, and Sarmatians) once occupied vast reaches from the South Russian to the Trans-Caspian Steppes and from Eastern Anatolia across the Iranian Plateau and the Hindu Kush to the heart of Central Asia. The greatest cross-pollination happened during the period of Mughal rule (1526-1857 CE) in India.

The first Mughal emperor, Babur, was a Turkic chieftain from modern-day Uzbekistan. He enlisted the help of the Iranian Safavid dynasty and Turkish Ottomans to aid his conquest of India. Due to the shared Islamic religion and the allegiances created by Babur, many Iranian wrestlers were brought to the Mughal court over the centuries. This was where the greatest cross-cultural exchange between the *zurxāne* and the *akhara* took place. It is to this period where many of the contentious techniques and tools of strength belong.

"While I seem on earth, abiding with you in the house, I ascend like Saturn to the seventh heaven." Jalāl al-Dīn Muḥammad Rūmī, Masnavi 2.16

It is no coincidence that the push-up board found in Iran is more common in western India, in the old Islamic Dekkan, than in eastern India. It is similarly interesting that many of the *mugdar* clubs of this eastern region of India tend to be smaller and shaped similarly to Iranian *mil*. The *mugdar* has a longer traceable history than the Iranian *mil*, suggesting it may have been used in India earlier than Iran.

The word *talīm* is used in the Maharashtra region of western India – a loan from the Iranian *ta'līm xāne* (house of instruction). Even the word *pahalwān* – used by the Indians for a wrestler or someone who trains in the *akhara* – is from the Iranian *pahlavān*. Up until 1947, the wrestling champion of India was called *"Rustam-i Hind"* (Rostam of India), another loan from Iran – Rostam is the main hero of Iranian epic.

"Do not imagine that the Way is short; vast seas and deserts lie before His court. Consider carefully before you start." Farīd ud-Dīn 'Aṭṭār, Conference of the Birds

WarYoga seeks to rediscover and reinvigorate the entire Indo-European metaphysical martial tradition without concern for petty squabbling between the various branch cultures. They all come from the same roots and branch off from the same great and noble trunk.

The WarYogin draws from the deep and ancient well of the Indo-Europeans, regardless of the small differences in the composition of the holy water. Indian, Iranian, Greek, Roman, Germanic, Slavic, and Celtic branches each have their own specialities and strengths, offering something of value to the WarYogin who seeks to reconnect and revive the ancient practices for his needs in this current age.

What follows is the second instalment of the great and sacred martial path of the Indo-European people. It is the path of holy war between Light and Darkness. There is no room for grey in the Iranian vision, just a simple choice as to which side of the fight each man will take.

For the WarYogin, the choice is clear. He is here to fight for the Light – for Right, for Good, for Truth.

"He created the righteous men to destroy and make powerless the Evil Spirit and all the demons." Bundahišn 1A.4

The Indo-Iranian Cosmos

"I will tell forth of the two Wills at the world's beginning, of who the Bounteous one speaks thus to the Hostile one: 'Neither our thoughts, nor our pronouncements, nor our intellects, nor our choices, nor our words, nor our deeds, nor our moralities, nor our souls are in accord.'" Yasna 45.2

Before the creation of the Cosmos, void separated Light and Darkness. The universe was created in seven stages. First sky, then water, earth, *haoma* (primal plant), bull (primal animal), Gayō Marətan (primal human), and fire. The origin of this creation and whether it had a creator was of no concern to the early Indo-Iranians.

Later, the Iranians believed that the spirit of the Darkness, Aṅgra Mainyu (or Ahriman), noticed the Light and attacked it, starting the eternal Cosmic battle between the two opposing forces. In order to beat Ahriman, the spirit of the Light, Ahura Mazdā (or Ohrmazd), created the Cosmos as a trap in which Darkness could be defeated.

"We worship the Fravaši of righteous Gayō Marətan, who first listened to the thought and teachings of Ahura Mazdā, from whom Mazdā fashioned forth the families of the Aryan peoples, the seed of the Aryan peoples." Fravardīn Yašt 13.87

Originally the universe was static, then the first plant (*haoma*), the first animal (bull) and the first human (Gayō Marətan/Gayōmard or Yima/Jamšid) were sacrificed and their seed dispersed, setting the cycle of death and rebirth in motion, and creating the multitudes of life from their original unity.

The Cosmic Maṇḍala is positioned centrally between the dark Lower Waters and the light Upper Waters. These are also expressed as Lower Chaos and Upper Chaos. The Cosmos is a sphere that is separated from the two Chaoses by *Asman* ("stone"), the stone vault of the heavens: the sky. Sky appears to the inhabitants of the Cosmos as a stone vault – an inverted bowl. The earth floats as a disc on the Cosmic Ocean *Vourukaša*.

"The sea Vourukaša is the gathering place of the waters, rising up and going down, up the aerial way and down the earth, down the earth and up the aerial way." Vīdēvdāt 21.4

This disc is surrounded by a ring in the Cosmic Mountain Range *Harā Bərəzaitī*. The *Vourukaša* also fills the ring, and on it are seven *kešvars* ("climes") or islands. In the East is *Savahi*; the *kešvar* in the West is *Arezahi*. The Southern *kešvars* are *Fradadhafšu* and *Vidadhafšu*. The Northern *kešvars* are *Vourubarešti* and *Vourjarešti*. *Xvaniratha* is the largest, central, and most important – bigger than the other six combined. They are surrounded and divided by the *Vourukaša* ocean.

Xvaniratha is where the central Cosmic Mountain – also *Harā Bərəzaitī* (or *Harburz/Hara*) – rises from the earth's centre, piercing the heavens. The Celestial River *Arədvī* flows down it and the sun, moon, and stars revolve around it. Located in Heaven, the waters of the Cosmic Ocean flow down the Cosmic Mountain's sacred rivers into the sea, from whence they flow back into the Cosmic Ocean. *Xvaniratha* is where the sacred *White Haoma* plant grows, and from where the Tree of Many Seeds scatters its medicinal germ into the world.

"And in its vicinity the tree was produced which is the White Haoma, the counteractor of decrepitude, the reviver of the dead, and the immortaliser of the living." Wizīdagīhā ī Zādspram 8.5

Xvaniratha is also the location of *Aryāna Vaējah*, the "Cradle of the Aryans." This "Expanse of the Aryans" is where the *Kayānids* (legendary hero kings) were created. *Aryāna Vaējah* is the place of the liturgies of Ahura Mazdā. It is the place where the first king Yima built the *vara*, where the elite shelter to repopulate the world after the Cosmic Winter. This *vara* is illuminated by its own light – an "inner light." *Xvaniratha* is the sacred island in the Cosmic Centre and seat of the Pole.

The Iranian Cosmos is comprised of three levels. Earth is holy, but the realm of mundane humanity. Atmosphere touches earth and the vault of the heavens; it is filled with potent forces that are ever changing. It surrounds man and is the arena of violent and awesome powers like the wind. Heaven is beyond the sphere of ordinary man – it is the place of transcendence. Sky gods in the heavens create and watch.

"The sky is made from the substance of the bloodstone, such as they also call diamond." Dādestān-ī Mēnōg ī Xrad 9.7

Traditionally in the Indo-Iranian pantheon, sky gods represented the priestly caste, atmospheric gods the martial caste, and feminine earth gods the pastoral caste. Mithra is a sky god, originally a priestly deity. Vayu is an atmospheric god: a warrior. Atmospheric gods live in the sky or on the Cosmic Mountain. The Sky gods are on its uppermost peak, the Emerald Keystone which penetrates the heavenly vault. Fire occupies all three levels.

In a late Zoroastrian creation text the *Bundahišn*, the sky has seven levels. These are, in ascending order, the cloud station, the firmament of the stars, the unmixable stars, the paradise where the moon resides, "infinite light" where the sun resides, the place of the Amahraspands (archangels), and the Throne of Ohrmazd (Ahura Mazdā). Later Iranian Ṣufīc thought built on this, considering the eighth *kešvar* to be the Emerald Peak of Cosmic Mountain, the threshold to the ninth sphere – the "Sphere of Spheres."

"The divine power is very superior to the strength of the Adversary ... The sunlight is far more powerful than the darkness." Dēnkard 3.329

Aside from being tripartite, the Indo-Iranian Cosmic structure is dualistic. The Cosmos is a fortress of Order surrounded by the dark waters of Chaos. This is a vertical differentiation: waters surrounding the heavens are a source of *Aša* ("Truth"), while those surrounding and below earth are sources of *Druj* ("Falsehood"), the anticosmic principle.

In later thought, the Upper Light is good, and the Lower Dark is evil: heavenly and infernal. Beyond the vault of heaven is the realm of the "Endless Lights," while below the earth is the realm of Darkness and Chaos. There was not such a severe demarcation in the original formation, and *Aša* and *Druj* were not considered as black and white, good and evil.

"Within time darkness is the opponent of light." Škand Gumānīg Wizār 9.16

Upper Chaos is the realm of Essence, of unmanifested possibilities. Lower Chaos is Substance: infinite possibilities. The divine acts as a barrier against the Chaos outside the Cosmos. Chaos, pure undifferentiated being, contains the germs of all possibilities – good as well as evil. Under the care of Ahura Mazdā, *Aša* ("Truth" or "Cosmic Order") is associated with fire and has its seat in the celestial waters. Truth, like Falsehood, emerges from Chaos.

Man is in the centre, median between two poles of the axis mundi. Man may choose to live under the dominion of Light or Darkness. To the unenlightened man, pure being is Chaos: a terrifying, but attractive state. To the mystic, pure being is the ultimate goal – beyond all opposites. This finds expression in the vertical differentiation of chaos.

"But man is more than a mirror to the Divine; in a very profound sense he is, at least potentially, pillar of the worlds. That is, in him all Creation is reflected – which means he can travel to both the subhuman and supra-human realms." Arthur Versluis, Song of the Cosmos

The magician who goes beyond can draw from the Upper Chaos and create his own Cosmos. Truth rises through the waters of Chaos, while Falsehood sinks. The WarYogin rises to the surface with Truth, while his eternal adversaries descend into the dark murk.

This Cosmic schema is not tied to any physical, manifest geography. It is the subtle spiritual landscape. The Indo-Iranian cosmos is the maṇḍala – it presents a meditative cosmology that leads the WarYogin back to the Centre: the Origin, the Exegesis, *ta'wil*, the Return.

The space between "this earth" and "that heaven" is bridgeable not only by the means of fire extant in each level, but also the Cosmic Mountain *Harā Bərəzaitī*. This is the path of communication between the levels: the avenue of transcendence.

"The spirit of the sky… accepted its role to be an enduring fortress against the Evil Spirit, preventing him from scurrying away in defeat." Bundahišn 1A.7

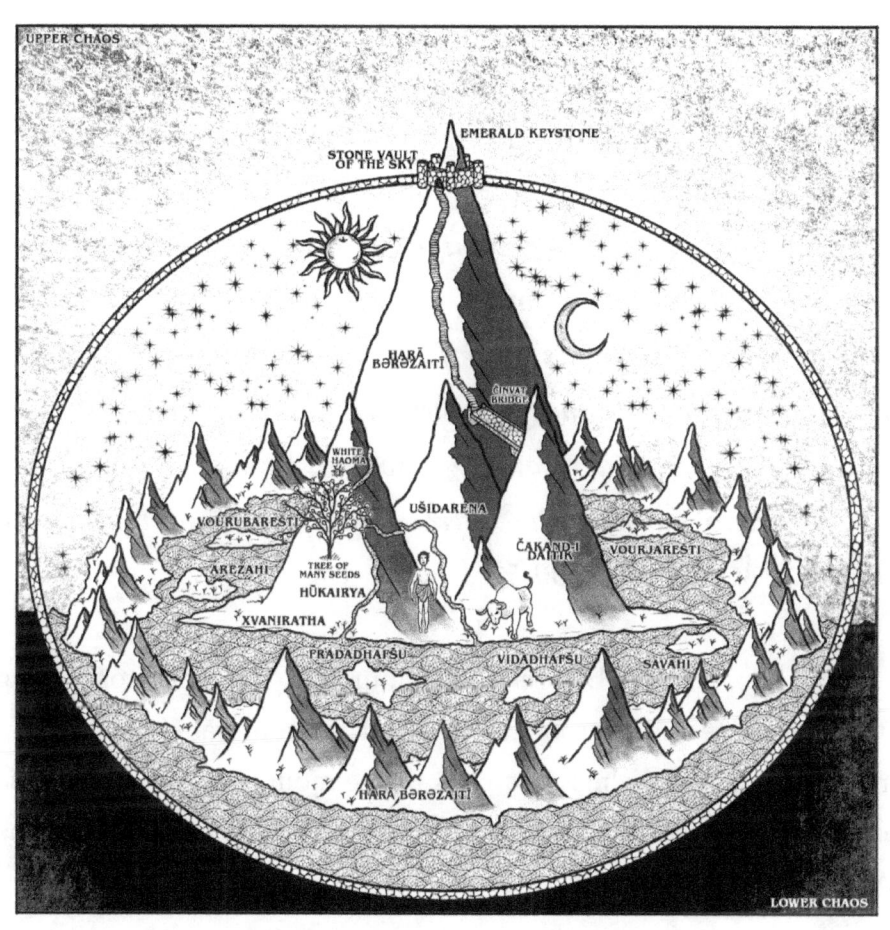

The Indo-Iranian Cosmos

The Celestial Mountain

"We worship Mithra... for whom the creator, Ahura Mazdā, fashioned a dwelling on top of shining lofty Harā which has many spurs, where there is no night of darkness, no cold nor hot wind, no illness causing much death, no defilement caused by the daēvas; nor do mists issue forth from lofty Haraitī; which all the Beneficent Immortals built in harmony with the sun, believingly, with understanding, thought, from a trusting mind, for him who surveys the entire material world from lofty Haraitī." Mihr Yašt 10.50-51

Harā Bərəzaitī is the Celestial Mountain, the Pole connecting planes of existence. It is rooted in the dark infernal states, reaching up into the aethereal realms. The peak of the mountain, the *taēra*, is the emerald keystone in the celestial vault. It is the point where the WarYogin can exit the material spheres into the immaterial strata.

The Iranian tradition clearly plots out the Indo-European Polar Mountain. There are three lower peaks below the highest level of *Harā Bərəzaitī*. First is *Hūkairya* ("Hugar the Very High"), as high as the stars. Down it flow the heavenly waters of *Arədvī Sūrā Anāhitā*, the Celestial River. Around this Water of Life grow marvellous plants, including *Gaokarena*, known also as "*White Haoma*." Next to *White Haoma* grows the Tree of Many Seeds that cures all ills.

This "Tree of Life" is common to all Indo-European traditions. In Iran it became the cypress tree, represented in Persian art as the *boteh* (paisley) pattern. The cypress is evergreen; it lives a long life and is strong yet flexible, making it a symbol of immortality. The Haoma is the lunar "tree," and the Tree of Many Seeds is solar.

"This is the sun track; and those are the souls who, in the world, exercised good sovereignty and rulership and chieftainship." Ardā Wīrāz-Nāmag 9.6

Next to *Hūkairya* is *Ušidarena* ("Ruby Mountain of the Dawns"), the peak first to be lit by auroral fires. The Celestial River passes from *Hūkairya* to *Ušidarena* and flows into *Vourukaša*, the Cosmic Ocean. If *Ušidarena* is the peak of the dawn and rebirth, then *Čakad-i Daītik* ("Peak of Judgement") is the dusk. It is the location of the *Činvatō Pərətu* ("Requiter's Crossing"), or more simply *Činvat Bridge*. Protected by two dogs, this is the bridge of judgement over which all souls must pass in order to be ruled on by the god Mithra and his two attendants Rašnu and Sraoša.

The righteous rejoin the pieces of their manifold soul and pass over the bridge, while the wicked fall to *Dušox* and *Hammistagān* (the infernal realms). The bridge and its three steps (*Humat* Star Station, *Hūxt* Moon Station, and *Huwaršt* Sun Station) links *Čakad-i Daītik* to the Cosmic Mountain of the Emerald Peak: the highest peak of *Harā Bərəzaitī*. The ascent of this mountain leads to *Garōdəmāna* ("House of

Song"), or *asar-rōšnīh* ("realm of light") the Throne of Ahura Mazdā. The Infinite Lights of *Garōdəmāna* (known also as *Garōtmān*) are the highest heaven available to the faithful of Zoroastrianism.

"The Daitih peak is in Airan-vej, in the middle of the world; reaching unto the vicinity of that peak is that beam-shaped spirit, the Činwad bridge, which is thrown across from the Alburz enclosure back to the Daitih peak." Dādēstān ī Dēnīg 21.2

The Celestial Mountain is the Pole. The mountain-axis is the axis of the worlds. It is the vertical route connecting the states of Being. The Celestial Mountain breaches the Celestial Vault through the Sun Door, the upward gate which passes beyond the House of Mithra and the Throne of Ahura Mazdā.

Having already reconstituted his tripartite Spirit, the WarYogin ascends the Holy Mountain, crosses the Bridge of Judgement to the Emerald Peak, and escapes the stone vault of heavens through the Sun Door. He travels past the Realm of Endless Lights, to the primordial state beyond the gods, beyond Ohrmazd's manifested creation, beyond Ahriman's dark influence to original pure Being. There he occupies the centre the Wheel of Time from where he sees all things unfolding, being created and destroyed, given manifest form and returned to formlessness.

"Do not stray from the straight path." Inscription of Darius I at Naqš-e Rostam

The Old Gods

"I am called Watcher, I am called Pursuer, I am called Creator, I am called Guardian, I am called Protector, I am called Knower." Yašt 1.13

To gain a clearer view of the Iranian gods, it is necessary to pull back and look at a wider view of Indo-Iranian and Indo-Aryan religion. Before sweeping into northern India and the Iranian plateau, these people were a single group sharing a religion and pantheon.

In India the Vedic religion developed, while the same gods took on different names and roles in Iran. The *ahuras* ("lords") were older gods; the daēvas ("shining ones") were upstarts. Originally, both priestly *ahuras* and martial *daēvas* (Vedic *asuras* and *devas*) were worshipped. In Iran, all gods were referred to as *yazatas*, a generic phrase meaning "deity." In the early Indic *ṚgVeda* both sets of gods work together against the demons (*dānavas*/*dasyus*).

"Likewise, the work manifested by him in the world – which is man – is in the likeness of these four classes of the world. As unto the head is priesthood, unto the hand is warriorship, unto the belly is husbandry, and unto the foot is artisanship." Škand Gumānīg Wizār 1.20-24

Like priests, *ahuras* used magical powers to intervene in the world. Favoured by warriors, *daēvas* were characterised by their strength and moral ambiguity. Both sets of gods were worshiped until one was demonised. In Vedic India warrior *devas* were favoured, whereas in Iran the priestly *ahuras* assumed the role of the good gods.

The Indians vilified asuras, including the great Vedic gods Varuṇa and Mitrá. In Iran, the *daēvas* became evil. During the tumultuous 2nd millennium BCE, both Indo-Aryan and Indo-Iranian branches of the Indo-European tribes militarised their pantheons, setting up gods to aid them in warfare, regardless of their original roles. The Iranians transformed their priestly *ahuras* into warlike deities, with Mithra becoming a strong warrior.

"The blood of the heroes is closer to God than the ink of the philosophers and the prayers of the faithful." Julius Evola, Metaphysics of War

Before their gods the *Arya* were neither fearful, nor servile. They believed themselves to be of the same blood as the gods: the blood of heroes. They did not propitiate demons like the tribes of their enemies, but supplied their gods with offerings in order that they had the strength to fight their adversaries.

They worshipped the sky, the sun, lightning, water, wind, and the Light. They upheld Order against the demons of Darkness, drought, and Chaos. They believed there was an eternal combat waged between the Gods of Light and the Forces of Darkness.

Ahuras

"I invoke the endless and sovereign Light. I invoke the bright, blissful Paradise of the Holy Ones." Vīdēvdāt 19.35-36

In the Iranian religion, *ahuras* were aligned with *Aša* (Truth/Order) and the *daēvas* with *Druj* (Lie/Disorder). Originally, the ahuric trinity of Ahura Mazdā, Mithra, and Vourunā (Apąm Napāt) were chief gods among the *Arya* of Iran. These three are the only gods given the lordly *ahura* title.

This trinity developed from the Indo-Aryan dual gods of order Mitrá and Varuṇa. Apąm Napāt is the name given to the god originally called Vourunā. Ahura Mazdā ("Wise Lord") was initially an epithet of Vourunā, but became a deity in his own right, eventually being uplifted to the head of the pantheon and possessor of *xšthra* (power/dominion).

While the *daēvas* were demonised by the Mazdāists, *daēva* worship continued to be practiced in some parts of Iran, particularly Sogdiana and Māzandarān, until the advent of Islam. Mazdāism became the main religion, and for the majority of Iranians the *daēvas* were seen as the bad gods. Indara (Vedic Indra) is therefore in the demonology of the Avestan *Vīdēvdāt*.

Daēvas

"I drive away Indara, I drive away Saurva, I drive away the daēva Nånhaithya." Vīdēvdāt 10.9

In most cases *daēva* means non-*ahura*. It is in this sense that, in the later Avesta, ancient gods are designated as *daēvas*: namely Indara, Saurva (Vedic Śarva, another name of Rudra), and Nånhaithya (Vedic Nāsatya, an epithet of the Aśvins). *Daēva* also designates demons, which were not formerly gods. Examples of these are Aēšma ("Wrath"), Druj ("Lie"), Apaoša ("Drought"), and Gaṇdarəwa (Vedic Gandharva). These *daēvas* were another class of beings that existed beside the *asuras* and the other *daēvas* in the early Indo-Iranian period.

Dahāka, like the Vedic Vṛtra, was the demonic serpent or dragon with three heads. He offered sacrifice to the water goddess Anāhitā to save himself, but he was defeated by Thraētaona. Gaṇdarəwa, was associated with water and slain by Kərəsāspa on the shore of Lake *Vourukaša*.

Aside from these two, Indara, Saurva, and Nånhaithya are the only demons to have a traceable Indo-Iranian origin. The rest of the demonic forces were a later development.

Sacrifice

"And we sacrifice to that better path that leads to that Best World." Visperad 7.2

Regardless of which set of gods were worshipped, the ancient Iranians built no temples and carved no idols. *Yasna* ("sacrifice") – particularly to the fire – was central to their religion, as it was to the Vedic Indians. The word *yasna* derives from *yaz*, meaning "to worship," which is also the root of *yazata* ("one worthy of sacrifice"). The sacrifice of *haoma*, bull, and human were all reenactments of the original sacrifice. They made the profane sacred and restored the Cosmos to its pristine condition.

This sacrifice happened on the mountaintops. It was not until the fourth century BCE that they built mountain-peak fire temples called *atash-gah*. The central sacrifice was that of the *haoma* libation (Vedic *soma*).

As in India, the *haoma* ritual became so complex that priests were required in order for it to be performed. Originally, the priestly class were not needed as it was simple, but over time only priests had the sacred knowledge of *mąthra* ("mantra") and *yasna*.

"Quickly cut out the sacrificial portion of the cow for swiftest Haoma, lest Haoma bind you." Hōm Yašt, Yasna 10.7

The *haoma* being poured into the fire recreated the primal unity before the sacrifice sundered the Cosmos apart. It united time and space, restoring balance. In pre-Zoroastrian Iran, the primordial man and king Yima was the sacrifice (he was later supplanted in this role by Gayō Marətan and others). The *daēvas* sacrificed Yima, cutting him up and rendering apart the original unity.

Gayō Marətan (also known as Gayōmard) means "mortal life." This abstraction was perhaps an epithet of Yima, as he was also considered a first king and held the title *garšah* ("King of the Mountain"). Humanity began with a single individual who was immortal, perfect, and beyond all dualities. Gayō Marətan, the "righteous," was rendered into the mortal human race through his sacrifice by the *daēvas* (later by Ahriman).

"When the peoples of evil kingdoms are deformed by the training in the false religion and guide themselves by the light of this false faith, then they spread immorality. And the earth becomes desolate, its inhabitants lead wicked lives, suffer pain, lose dignity through evil intentions, become destitute, and owing to wickedness appear of evil mien." Dēnkard 3.347

This religion was that of Indo-European cattle raiders. In this violent and volatile world existed several categories of holy man. The *āthravan* (Vedic *atharvan*) was the fire priest, responsible for keeping the sacred flame alive. The *zaotar* (Vedic *hotṛ*) was the libation priest who performed the most important function of pouring *haoma* on the fire.

The *stator* (Vedic *stotṛ*) was the eulogist; the *ərəši* (Vedic *ṛṣi*) was a poet seer. The *kavi* was a magician with knowledge of magic and immortality. The warriors were accompanied on their raids by the *usig*, a warrior shaman who pitched magical battle.

These raiders degenerated into orgiastic rowdies. The world became more chaotic. *Aša* (Order) gave way to *Druj* (Disorder). A *zaotar* of the priestly caste Zarathuštra Spitāma reacted to this, changing the world forever.

"Give unto that man brightness and glory, give him health of body, give him sturdiness of body, give him victorious strength of body, give him full welfare of wealth, give him a virtuous offspring, give him long, long life, give him the bright, all-happy, blissful abode of the Holy Ones." Ohrmazd Yašt 1.33

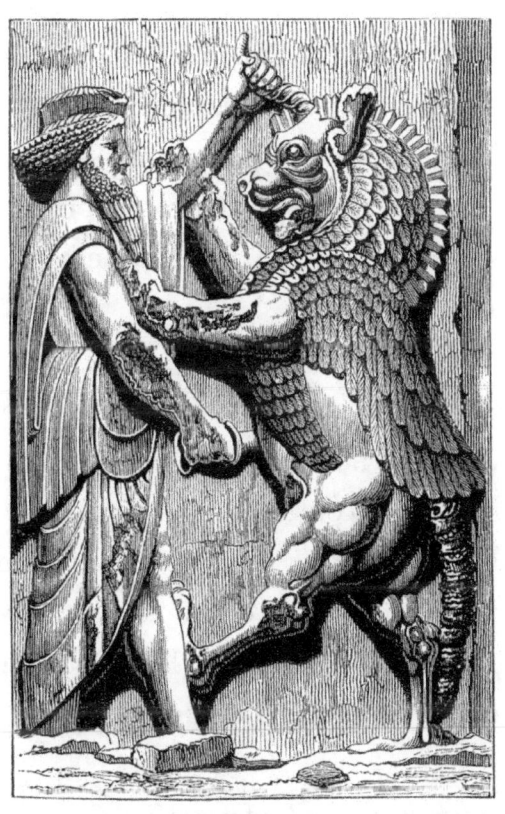

"The King Killing Angra Mainyu" Relief, Persepolis

Zarathuštra

"This man here I have found, the only one who listens to Our teachings: Zarathuštra Spitāma. He desires, mindful, on Our behalf and Right's, to broadcast Our praises, as I harness his well-constructed utterance." Yasna 29.8

The figure of Zarathuštra Spitāma – later called Zartošt and known to the Greeks as Zoroaster – is a mysterious one. Aged thirty, the priest Zarathuštra received a pure-light vision of the god Ahura Mazdā while in a river fetching water for a spring ceremony. Very little is known about the man and his life, whether he existed, and if so, when and where.

Persian historical sources at the time of the Achaemenid Dynasty of Darius and Xerxes do not mention Zarathuštra (a name meaning "Camel Driver"), but contemporary Greek sources talk of "Zoroaster." Outside the Greek material, all that remains connected to Zarathuštra are religious texts of the Zoroastrian faith. With one notable exception, these are of a much later date, though may have been transmitted orally from high antiquity.

"He who among mortals has gratified Spitāma Zarathuštra by his concern, that man is worthy of renown." Yasna 46.13

The oldest part of the *Avesta*, the holy cannon of Zoroastrianism, are the *Gāthās*. These too were not committed to paper for many centuries, but were preserved for two millennia through the memorised oral tradition. Composed in an archaic northern tongue, the hymns are impenetrable in the extreme. Both language and content point to the ancient North – possibly dating them to the 14th century BCE (contemporary with the Indic *Vedas*) and positioning them geographically in northeastern Greater Iran. This was a land of pastoralism and the three Indo-European castes: *āthravan* (priests), *arthaeštar* (warriors) who also formed the *xšathra* (ruling class), and the *vāstryōfšugant* (cattlemen).

These hymns are spoken in the first-person from the mouth of Zarathuštra. They differ from the later Zoroastrian religion in many regards, particularly due to their devotion to one god and his archangels to the exclusion of all others. This god, Ahura Mazdā, may already have been part of the Iranian pantheon as part of the Old Persian religion, which sprung forth from the Indo-Iranian religion.

"Good Thought, and the souls of the righteous, the Reverence, with which are Piety and Libation, besides... that confers lasting dominion." Yasna 49.10

The different nature of the Gāthic material to the rest of the *Avesta* has led many to categorise the original religion of Zarathuštra as Zarathuštrianism, distinct from the later Zoroastrianism that developed from it. Zoroastrianism is the fusion of the old Iranian religion – which never lost popularity – and Zarathuštrianism. The

Gāthās are the only part of the *Avesta* considered Zarathuštrian. The rest, the "*Younger Avesta,*" is Zoroastrian. The *Gāthās* are focussed on ethical dualism centred around the deity Ahura Mazdā.

The Bronze Age steppe saw an increase in raiding culture and the professional warband. Zarathuštra saw this as an unacceptable attack on herders and traditional order. The Avestan term *mairyō* (Vedic *márya*) meaning warrior, specifically the youthful wolf warrior, came to be a pejorative term in Iran. It was replaced in India with *kṣatriya* ("one with power") and in Avestan culture with *arthaēštar* ("one standing in a chariot").

"Among wolves, there is a greater need to smite the two-legged than the four-legged one." Fragment from the Artēštārestān

The poets of the *R̥gVeda* lauded the *márya*, while Zarathuštra branded them as scoundrels, making their main deity Indra the greatest of the *daēvas*. The *mairyō* were attached to the cult of the gods Mithra and Vərəthragna. The Vedic material relishes the cattle raid, while the Gāthic denounces it.

Iranian texts condemn the "two-legged *mairyō* and four-legged wolves," sometimes referring to the youth warband as "two-legged wolves." A fragment of the *Artēštārestān* (a lost Avestan military manual preserved in the *Dēnkard* 8.26) confirms the Zarathuštrian distaste for raiders. Following the Zoroastrian reform, the Indo-Iranian youth warbands were demonised, and heroes such as the *männerbund* archetype Kərəšaspa lost their importance and prestige.

"They set me apart from the clan and tribe; I am not pleased with the communities I consort with, nor with the region's wrongful rulers." Yasna 46.1

Aēšma (later a name of the demon Wrath) is the state of furor that warriors cultivated for battle – also called "fury." In a heightened state of wolfish rage induced by partaking the *haoma* draft, the youthful *mairyō* entered the battle to defeat their foes and steal their cattle. The Scythian *Saka Haumavarga* ("Haoma-wolves") tribe personified this wolfish warrior tendency among the Indo-European neighbours of the Iranian people centuries after they had ceased to practice raid culture themselves.

Zarathuštra likely experienced first-hand the attack of professional warriors and saw it as a "wicked" attack on the established order of his pastoral society. It is against this backdrop that Zarathuštra, after receiving a divine revelation, set out to create a revised religion with a monotheistic tendency. He focussed his new religion on Ahura Mazdā ("Wise Lord") and his dark opponent Angra Mainyu ("Hostile Spirit").

"There are two Wills, the twins who in the beginning made themselves heard though dreaming, those two kinds of thought, of speech, of deed, the better and the evil; between them the well-doers discriminate rightly, but ill-doers do not." Yasna 30.3

The religious reform of Zarathuštra consisted only in promoting ethical conversion: that is by insisting on the necessity of choosing good and renouncing evil. It didn't annihilate the Iranian polytheistic religion. Although it appears that Northeastern Iran may have taken up the religion of Zarathuštra during the prophet's lifetime.

His religious "reform" was that of the priestly *zaotar* against the raiding warriors. He saw the cattle raids as *Druj* ("Lie") taking over from *Aša* ("Truth" or "Order"). This is the opposite side of the religious coin from the ṚgVedic warriors of Indra righteously raiding the southern *dāsas* ("slaves").

"This, that I may overcome all those who are hostile to, of daēvas and mortals, and sorcerers and witches, tyrants, Kavis, Karapans, and two-footed scoundrels, deceivers of truth and four-footed wolves, and the broad fronted daēvic army, flying demons." Hōm Yašt 9.18

As the warrior bands were at the core of the prophet's reforms, he strongly opposed two vital parts of the warrior ritual: cow sacrifice and the consumption of *haoma*. He was unable to stop them since they were deeply ingrained into the Indo-European psyche, but he attempted to change the way they were viewed. The cow was still the most sacred animal, so Zarathuštra did not exclude it from sacrifice – only from sacrifice to *daēvas*.

Haoma was drunk by warriors but administered by priests. Zarathuštra demonised *haoma* as it was specifically important to

Indara, a *daēva* he particularly despised. However, the central ritual of the Zoroastrian cannon, the *yasna*, is still to this day a *haoma* sacrifice. Zarathuštra spoke out against the other priests, particularly two classes who aided the cattle raiding warriors: *kavis* and *karapans*.

Ahura Mazdā

"May Ohrmazd give thee the august rank and throne of a champion!" Šayest Na-Šayest 22.1

Pre-Zarathuštrian Iran had already shown a preference for worshipping *ahuras*, the older gods, over *daēvas*. Zarathuštra emphasised this rift and demonised the *daēvas* further. He elevated Ahura Mazdā as he had a personal connection to him following a vision he had.

This prompted him to start his religious crusade. While Mazdā may have ascended prior to the time of Zarathuštra, it was the prophet who gave him the previously unassigned role of creator.

Mazdāism worshipped one god called Ahura Mazdā, later called Ohrmazd in Old Persian. The traditional Indo-Iranian religion had at its head the pair of gods Vourunā and Mithra. Zarathuštra amalgamated the concepts of Mithra-Vourunā into Mazdāism.

"Indo-Iranian heritage can be glimpsed through cracks in the Zoroastrian facade." Jaan Puhvel, Comparative Mythology

The "Wise Lord" Ahura Mazdā was a development from Vourunā (Vedic Varuṇa), with some elements of the Sky Father Dyaoš (Vedic Dyáuṣ) also incorporated. Ahura Mazdā was originally an epithet which became the name of the god. Vourunā, or Ahura Mazdā, is the Iranian counterpart of Vedic Varuṇa. In the ṚgVeda 1.24.14, Varuṇa is also invoked as the Wise Lord (Asura Pracatáḥ).

Only Ahura Mazdā and Varuṇa are the object of intense personal religious experience in the Indo-Iranian and Indo-Aryan traditions. Mazdā's element is *ātar* ("fire") in Avestan lore. This is a divergence from Varuṇa whose element is water. Fire more properly belongs to the *ahura* Mithra. Ahura Mazdā was originally the god of the Celestial Chaotic Waters in which Truth is found.

"But may that man attain yet better than the good, who should teach us the straight paths of advancement in this material existence and that of thought, the true gradients that Ahura inhabits." Yasna 43.3

Like Varuṇa, Mazdā tends to Cosmic Order: *Aša* (Vedic *Ṛta*). This is Truth as a Cosmic power. Mazdā is father of Aša. Zarathuštra made Truth an emanation of Ahura Mazdā, but Truth is primordial and in both pre and post-Zarathuštrian religion.

Aša and Druj

"The way to that true service is known through wisdom, is believed through truth, and is utilised through goodness; and

the path of excellence more particularly leads to it." Dādēstān ī Dēnīg 7.6

Zarathuštra attempted to amalgamate monotheism with dualism. While syncretising Mazdāism and Indo-Iranian religion, he added that alongside primordial Truth existed Falsehood. He also introduced human choice and a struggle between good and evil into Iranian religion. He properly set up the dualism of *Aša* ("Truth" and "Order") and *Druj* ("Lie," "Disorder," and "Calamity"), polarising these ancient concepts and making them pivotal to his new religion.

Zarathuštra took the latent dualism between *Aša* and *Druj*, turning it into a clear dualism fought on the battleground of Earth, where each human must choose a side. The prophet stated that man must choose between Truth and Falsehood – that transcendence lies in his own choices.

"May we be the ones who will make this world splendid, Mindful One and Ye Lords, bringers of change, and Right, as our minds come together where insight is fluctuating." Yasna 30.9

Zarathuštra's expressions of religion had an ethical, Cosmic dualism. It was only in later Zoroastrianism it became simply good versus evil. He set the poles of his dualism in the world of *Aša* (purity, Right, Cosmic Order) and *Druj* (pollution, disorder, calamity), dividing inhabitants of these two modes of existence as *Ašavan* ("Truth-Possessor") and *Drugvant* ("Lie-Possessor").

In Zarathuštra's pure doctrine there is a dualism between *Aša* and *Druj*, as well as Spənta Mainyu ("Beneficent Spirit") and Aŋgra Mainyu ("Hostile Spirit"). Aešma – the *mainyu* (spirit) of "fury" was elevated to represent the polar opposite of Ahura Mazdā's order. In the *Younger Avesta*, composed long after the death of Zarathuštra, Aešma is referred to as Aŋgra Mainyu; in the *Pahlavi* literature of later Zorostrianism he is called Ahriman.

"Of the two Spirits, the follower of the Lie chose the worst of actions, the most beneficent chose Truth." Yasna 30.5

Ahura Mazdā sired twin brothers: Spənta Mainyu and Aŋgra Mainyu. Both were distinguished in thought, word, and deed, but the first was good and the second wicked. Spənta Mainyu was the creative organ of Ahura Mazdā and was later absorbed into the singular godhead Ohrmazd. After this reabsorption, Ohrmazd directly opposes Ahriman himself.

Initially, Spənta Mainyu created on behalf of his father all that is good in the world, while Aŋgra Mainyu created all that is wicked, including the *daēvas* and *xrafstras* (noxious creatures). *Aša* and *Druj* were championed by Spənta Mainyu and Aŋgra Mainyu respectively.

"For then destruction will come upon Wrong's prosperity, and the swiftest steeds will be yoked from the fair dwelling of Vohu Manah, of Ahura Mazdā, and of Aša, and they will be winners in good repute." Yasna 30.10

Aside from the reassignment of old gods to demonic roles, and the personification of *Aša* and *Druj*, new abstractions came into existence through Zarathuštra: the *Aməša Spənta* (Beneficent Immortals). Spənta Mainyu was foremost of these seven angelic beings, who were not seen as gods in their own right. Monotheism was centred on Ahura Mazdā who emanated the seven *Aməša Spənta* (supernatural aspects of himself).

These in turn are the counterparts of the "elements" man, cattle, fire, metal, earth, water, and plants. Aside from Spənta Mainyu ("Beneficent Spirit"), they are: Vohu Manah ("Good Mind" or "Good Purpose" representing cattle), Aša Vasišta ("Best Truth" or "Righteousness" – fire), Xšathra Vairya ("Excellent Rulerdom" or "Desirable Dominion" – metal), Spənta Ārmaiti ("Right Thought," "Bounteous Harmony," or "Holy Devotion" – earth), Haurvatāt ("Wholeness," "Perfection," or "Health" – waters), and Amərətāt ("Deathlessness" or "Immortality" – plants).

"The Ohrmazdean essence is warm, humid, shining, fragrant, light, and visible from within." Bundahišn 26.131

If these are aspects of Ahura Mazdā, then so too must be Angra Mainyu. The creator draws order from chaos. In extracting the good aspects, he also pulls out the evil. These *Aməša Spənta* are good qualities that lie within man; they are representative of internal gods.

Spənta Ārmaiti is the higher inner voice. Xšathra Vairya is the aspiration that must be fought for. Aša Vasišta is inner order. Vohu

Manah is direction. Haurvatāt is the holistic method. Amərətāt is the diamond bodily vehicle. Also latent within man is the degenerative spirit of Aṇgra Mainyu.

While the concepts of Cosmic battle are ancient, Zarathuštra gave us the idea that we are soldiers due to our freewill. The Cosmic War is fought within the hearts and souls of men on the internal cosmic battlefield. Zarathuštra was the first to codify this Greater Holy War.

The battle of gods and spirits is within as well as without. The gods fight within the WarYogin. He is a warrior on the battlefield of Self. The ahuric doctrine of the WarYogin allows him to elevate his lordly traits in order to defeat the daēvic shortcomings that lie within.

"When he saw valour and victory greater than his own, he scurried back into the darkness and fabricated many demons, those destructive creatures hungry for battle." Bundahišn 1.16

Zoroastrianism

"Be it known that, men who live in this world with their minds devoted to the good religion, and who are equipped with sacred weapons, are victorious and powerful and conduce to the happiness of their fellows. Worthy efforts proceed from them in this world. They are the cause of the activity and prosperity of the world, and the guardians of its creatures." Dēnkard 3.268

The religion Zarathuštra hoped to establish did not succeed in ousting the old gods, but in the end absorbed them back into the fold. Zoroastrianism – the later version of Zarathuštrianism – made concessions to the Old Persian religion, allowing some of the more popular gods to be rehabilitated and repurposed. For example, Mithra transitioned from a god of the priestly caste to one of the warriors, taking over much of the role of the *daēva* Indara.

Zarathuštrianism was initially practiced in Eastern Iran outside the Persian Empire. This was the heartland of the faith until Cyrus II of Persia revolted against the Medes in 550 BCE, taking their empire and founding the Achaemenid (Old Persian: Haxāmanišyah) dynasty. Eastern Iran also fell to Cyrus the Great (Old Persian: Kūruš) in the middle of the 6th century BCE. This allowed the spread of Zoroastrian ideas, eventually to the later Achaemenid kings.

"Darius the king says: By the will of Ahuramazdā I am king. Ahuramazdā delivered the kingship to me." Inscription of Darius I at Behistun

Darius I (522 - 486 BCE) worshipped Ahura Mazdā publicly above all other gods, but his inscriptions mention the "other gods who are." He was devoted to "Ahuramazdā," but does not mention *Aša*, *daēvas*, the *Aməša Spənta*, nor Zarathuštra. Both the Great Kings Darius (Old Persian: Dārayavahuš) and Xerxes (Old Persian: Xšayāṛšā) probably practiced the Old Persian religion, which also uplifted Ahura Mazdā. There is no evidence either had knowledge of Zarathuštra.

Darius saw Ahura Mazdā, god of *Airyanəm Vaējah* ("Expanse of the Aryans" – then the name of Eastern Iran), as the unifying deity of the Iranians. He, a Persian, adopted this god as he continued to consolidate Iran. Iranian groups like the Persians and the Saka worshipped Mazdā without knowledge of Zarathuštra.

Darius installed Mazdāism (not Zarathuštrianism) as the religion of the state. His successor Xerxes (486-465 BCE) then condemned the worship of *daēvas* in his Daiwadāna inscription. Both Darius and Xerxes attributed to Ahura Mazdā their divine right to rule, styling themselves *Xšāyathiya Xšāyathiyānām* ("king of kings"), agent of Ahura Mazdā.

"And among these countries there was a place where previously false gods were worshipped. Afterwards, by the

favor of Ahuramazdā, I destroyed that sanctuary of the demons, and I made proclamation, 'The demons shall not be worshipped!'" Daēva Inscription of Xerxes at Persepolis

The Magi from Media and Western Iran were a class of professional priests who served any of the various cults of the time. They could sing a hymn to any deity and a sacrifice had to be performed in the presence of a Magus. The Magi of Darius and Xerxes were precursors to Zoroastrian priests.

The Magi learned of Ahura Mazdā to satisfy Darius and Xerxes. They performed the role required of their caste with the Zarathuštrian god, who was then foreign to them. Darius imposed his Mazdāism upon the Magian priesthood, which was suffering from royal disfavour in the wake of the insurrection of Gaumata the Magus.

The Magi took up Ahura Mazdā in addition to their pantheon, to whom they chanted theogonies. These became the precursors to the Zoroastrian *yašts* (hymns).

The Magi's powerful influence also spread east, bringing the old gods back into the Zarathuštrian religion. Soon after 441 BCE, the Zarathuštrian priests of *Airyanəm Vaējah* created Zoroastrianism from the disorganised fragments of the religion being practiced, bringing it back under their control. Zoroastrianism conceded the old Iranian deities (with some exceptions), subordinating them to Ahura Mazdā. This, the Zoroastrians saw as their way to spread their religion out of Eastern Iran.

"May Ahuramazdā, Anahita, and Mithra protect me from all evil, and that which I have built may they not shatter nor harm." Inscription of Artaxerxes II at Susa

By the reign of Artaxerxes II (404-359 BCE), an eclectic version of Zoroastrianism was adopted as the official state religion of the empire. However, the inscriptions of Artaxerxes (Old Persian: Artaxšaçah) specifically mention Mithra and Anāhitā. He encouraged the worship of the goddess through her images, which he spread throughout the empire.

The polytheistic religions of the various peoples of the empire were accepted, but Zoroastrianism was the religion of the elites, used to further their rule. Fire temples and the status of fire was elevated. It was in this period that *Nowruz*, the Festival of Fire at the spring equinox or Persian New Year, was instated.

Celebrating the temporary victory of Light over Darkness, it was the most important of the seven holy days, which reflected the seven aspects of the godhead Ahura Mazdā and seven stages of creation. This was also echoed through the seven-part worship of the *yasna*. Daily devotions (originally three times a day, then five) were done in the presence of sacred fire: either the sun or hearth.

"Darius the king says: He who worships Ahuramazdā will be blessed both living and dead." Inscription of Darius I at Behistun

In contrast to the Ahura Mazdā of Zarathuštra and Darius, the Ahura Mazdā of the *Younger Avesta* is a shadow of the Wise Lord. He retained his position at the head of the pantheon, but was sapped of all personality. Due to his abstract nature, Ahura Mazdā lost meaning to the point he became little more than an invocation. He became irrelevant to day-to-day religious concerns due to his lofty nature. This led to the *Younger Avesta* reinstatement of traditional gods.

The *yašts* (hymns) of the Younger Avesta are only superficially Zarathuštrian and their content is really Old Iranian and Indo-Iranian. The deities Mithra, Haoma, and Vayu (Vedic Mitrá, Soma, and Vāyū) from the Indo-Iranian tradition – alongside the Old Iranian gods Tištrya, Arədvī Sūrā Anāhitā, and the *Fravašis* – take the main stage.

"The business of the warriors is to defeat the enemy; and to keep their own country and land unalarmed and tranquil."
Dādestān ī Mēnōg ī Xrad 31.9-10

In 334 BCE, Alexander the Great crossed the Hellespont into Asia, launching his assault on the Persian Empire. By the end of 330 BCE, the Macedonian had burned the city of Persepolis to the ground; Darius III – last king of the Achaemenid dynasty – was dead, killed by his relative Bessus (Old Persian: Bayaça) who unsuccessfully attempted to seize the throne for himself under the title Artaxerxes V. Following 190 years of Hellenistic rule under the Argead and Seleucid dynasties, Persia was awash with foreign cults. The Mazdā cult became just one of many in a cosmopolitan religious landscape.

In 141 BCE, the Parthians (or Aškānī), invaded the Old Persian territory and overthrew the Greeks, ruling for almost four centuries. A more traditional Indo-European Scythian-Iranian group, they were more remote and decentralised. Their territory on the empire's steppe fringe meant they were removed from the Semitic religious influence of the Near East that had seeped into Iran. They worshipped Mithra, bringing the worship of this ancient Indo-European deity back to the fore of the elite religion. Their decentralisation meant there was no dominant priestly group: the warrior-kings led ritual, offering the bull sacrifice to their warrior god.

"I shall sacrifice to Mithra of wide cattle pastures, who has a thousand ears, ten thousand eyes. I shall sacrifice to his mace, well aimed against the skulls of the daēvas, Mithra of wide cattle pastures. And I shall sacrifice to that friendship which is the best of friendships, that between the Moon and the Sun." Khwaršed Niyayeš 15

It wasn't until the third century CE, under the Sasanians, that Mazdāism became dominant once more. In 226 CE the Persian Sasanians began their rule of four hundred years. For the first time since 331 BCE, a Persian king sat on the throne.

Naming their kingdom Ērānšahr (from Old Persian Aryāna Khašatra – "Aryan Imperium"), the Sassanid kings were sponsors of Mazdāism. They, like the Achaemenids, attributed their right to rule to Ahura Mazdā. The first Sassanid king Ardašir I had his image receiving the ring of rulership from Mazdā carved into the rock face of the ancient tombs at Persepolis, strengthening his connection not only to the god, but also to Darius and Xerxes.

Mazdāean priests became powerful, codifying the religion as that of the state. Under King Vahram I in 271 CE, the Zoroastrian high priest Kardīr crushed the other faiths with the king's blessing. He had the charismatic prophet Mānī killed, abolishing Manichaeism and making Mazdāism the official state religion.

"Be it known that light is of two kinds. One is the light of the vision of the physical eye, and thus it may be seen by the open eye of the body. The other is the light that is seen with the mind's eye and it is the knowledge perceived from the clear vision of the soul's eye." Dēnkard 3.250

Late in the Sassanid rule, the Magi began the painstaking process of collecting and recording oral prayers and formulas which had been passed down unwritten through the millennia. This comprehensive work was known as the *Avesta*. By the time the *Avesta* was written in the sixth century CE, much of it was no longer understood, similar the *ṚgVeda* in India.

The priests also wrote the *Zand*, a commentary on the ancient and incomprehensible prayers and hymns. Before this codification, a multitude of practices were used and *daēva* worship was common. The practice of "sorcerers" in the *Avesta* and *Pahlavi* books are much like those ascribed to Magi in general by Greco-Roman sources.

> "He is a complete defender of his own empire from opponents of a different nature, and his champions and troops become victorious in the struggle and contest. And in the end he is a bringer of victory to his own creatures, as regards every iniquity." Škand Gumānīg Wizār 12.61-63

Following incursions from the Byzantine Empire and civil war, the Sassanids fell to the Rashidun Caliphate in the mid-seventh century CE. With the coming of Islam, Zoroastrianism faded and much of the *Avesta* was corrupted and lost. Only five of the original twenty-one books of the Sassanid *Avesta* survive today.

Zurvān

> "From time he fashioned the firmament, the body of Zurvān of Long Dominion, Lord of Fate." Bundahišn 3.7

While no longer the main religion of Iran, Zoroastrianism remained in pockets of the country and developed further. Books called the *Pahlavi Texts* recorded rules of the religion and more complex mythology of later Zoroastrianism.

Ohrmazd (Ahura Mazdā) is pitted directly against Ahriman (Aŋgra Mainyu) rather than through his agent Spəṇta Mainyu, who the godhead has absorbed. Texts such as the 9th century *Bundahišn* set out this conflict with Ohrmazd, creating the world and finite time as a trap for Ahriman: a trap the anti-god entered through a hole in the celestial firmament. Ahriman can only fight within the temporal and spacial limits set forth by Ohrmazd as the battlefield, while the creator remains outside these constraints in infinite time and Light.

"He created all the creatures inside the sky, a stronghold, like a fortress in which are stored all the weapons needed for battle." Bundahišn 1A.7

While it is a late source, the *Bundahišn* (Book of Creation) is based on the lost *Dāmdād Nask* (Avestan Book of Creation). Its authors say it is sourced from the *dēn* (Avestan *daēnā*) which translates to "vision." The *daēnā* is the divine female counterpart who the male soul of the dead is joined by on the *Činvat Bridge* of judgement.

In the *Bundahišn*, Ahriman is not a product of the material world. His darkness invaded Ohrmazd's creation from the immaterial plane. The hostile spirit was trapped within material existence where he could be defeated by the good thoughts, words, and deeds of men. This is the *kārezār* ("battlefield") between forces of Light and Darkness. Mankind is able to choose which side they are fighting for through their ideas, speech, and actions.

"It happened to Ahriman, in the gloom and darkness, that he was walking humbly on the borders, and meditating other things he came up to the top, and a ray of light was seen by him; and because of its antagonistic nature to him he strove that he might reach it, so that it might also be within his absolute power." Wizīdagīhā ī Zādspram 1.1

Before the material world existed, there was an immaterial spiritual realm divided into Light and Darkness. Ahriman noticed the Light world of Ohrmazd and attacked it from his Dark realm. The two agreed to fight and Ohrmazd created the material world as the battlefield upon which Light would triumph. All creation makes up the field of battle: good stars versus evil planets, good animals against vermin, heroes versus witches and sorcerers.

The current time is the *Gumēzišn* ("Mixture") where both good and evil exist in the world. The world is also made up of *mēnōg* (intangible spiritual realm) and *gētīg* (tangible material realm). These two "creations" were once separate, but are now intermingled. This period is cognate to the Indic *Kali Yuga*: age of the demon Kali who will be defeated by Kalki, final avatar of the god Viṣṇu. Similarly, the forces of Ohrmazd will defeat those of Ahriman at the end of the *Gumēzišn* to bring about the *Vizarišn* ("Separation").

"At the Final Body, the creatures of Ohrmazd will have perfect power for ever and ever; that is infinity. And at that time, the creatures of Ahriman will be destroyed, so that the Final Body can come to be." Bundahišn 1.10

While this is seen as a certain victory in the Mazdāean branch of Zoroastrianism, in the Zurvānite branch it is not guaranteed and there is no final decisive battle. Since time is a prevalent theme in the *Bundahišn*, some scholars have taken this book to be evidence of a heretical cult called Zurvānism.

The tenth century epic *Šahnāme* (Book of Kings) has also been said to have Zurvānist influences. This is because it has the themes that fate is inevitable and both good and evil come from God. Zurvānism was possibly predominant in the early years of the Sassanid Dynasty, but everything about the cult is obscure.

Zurvānism and its key creation mythology are not mentioned directly in any Iranian sources, but are found in contemporary Greek, Syraic, Arabic, and Armenian works. The Zurvānist myth is most clearly described in the fifth century Armenian treatise *Refutation of the Sects* by the Christian writer Eznik of Kołb. Zurvān is god of *zamān* (time) and *bakt* (fate). In this tradition, he is the primordial deity from whom Ohrmazd and Ahriman emerge as twin brothers.

"They say that before there was anything, not heaven, or earth, or any creature in heaven or on earth, there was someone called Zurvan by name, which can be translated as fortune or glory. For a thousand years he made sacrifices that he might have a son, Ormizd by name, who would make heaven and earth and everything in them... And everything which Ormizd made was good and straight, while everything Ahriman made was evil and crooked." Eznik of Kołb, Refutation of the Sects 2.1

Zurvān wished for a son and performed sacrifices for a thousand years. He conceived Ohrmazd within himself, but then expressed doubt as to whether he had performed the sacrifices correctly. This doubt was the sin that allowed Ahriman to be conceived.

As Zurvān had promised dominion to his firstborn son, Ahriman fought his way out of his father's navel. He thus gained a nine thousand-year reign. Ohrmazd was born and was given the *barsom* (holy bundle) of priesthood.

In this quasi-fatalist school of thought, Ahriman currently reigns over the Cosmos. The forces of Ohrmazd must wage war against the *dēvs* (*daēvas*) and *druz* ("fiends") of Ahriman to try and gain victory in the Cosmic War – a war without certain victory for Ohrmazd. The traditional caste hierarchy is also made apparent in Zurvānism: Ohrmazd wears the priestly white clothing, Vay wears the warrior's red, and Zurvān wears the blue of the farmer.

"Vay's duty is removing evil from both Creations, for the Good Spirit created him in order to put an end to the Evil Spirit during the battle." Bundahišn 3.6

The wind god Vay (Vayu) is given a particular prominence as the warrior deity who will fight Ahriman directly in the Final Battle for the Cosmos. Vay is an ambiguous god with both light and dark traits. He forms part of the horde of the great god Mithra – the army of order that will march against the chaotic forces of Ahriman. The apocatastatic *Frašōkərəti* ("Making Gloriously Brilliant") is the Cosmic renewal: the return to order. In Mazdāism, the outcome is final and guaranteed; in Zurvānism, it is neither.

Time is cyclical: the forces of Light will ever be pitted against the armies of Darkness. Ahriman will always be forced back to his dark lair to lick his wounds, but he will again gather strength there. The WarYogin prepares to fight in the horde of Mithra alongside Vayu and the other warriors of the eternal god of Light. He does not withdraw into world-renouncing contemplation, but makes his ascesis one of action.

He fights his enemies without and within unrelentingly, zealously. Knowing he is surrounded, his victory over Darkness is never complete. The WarYogin seeks transcendence in order that he may become a powerful warrior of the Light.

"The world is filled with our adversaries and enemies, and all this realm is the abode of Ahriman." Šahnāme

Mithra

"With libations I shall worship the powerful god, strong Mithra, strongest in the world of creatures." Mihr Yašt 10.6

If any god can be seen as emblematic of the Iranians, it is Mithra. Despite Ahura Mazdā being at the head of the pantheon, Mithra – his counterpart and complimentary deity – was always more popular with the Iranian nobility. Mithrayazna ("Worship of Mithra") formed the esoteric religion of the Elite, with Mithra being referred to as *bagā vazrakā* ("great god").

Alongside Mazdāism, Mithraism was the older and possibly more popular religion among the entire population of the Iranian heartland. Cyrus the Great considered Mithra to be the supreme deity. Darius attributed his installation as king to being chosen by Mithra, who he claimed was the primordial ruler. Mithra was the family deity of the Achaemenid kings; more donations were made by them for Mithraic rituals than Mazdāean ones according to the palace records from Persepolis. The later Parthian rulers were primarily Mithraists also.

Zarathuštra sublimated Mithra's essence into Vohu Manah, but he came back in the *Yašts* of the *Younger Avesta*. Zoroastrian fire temples are still called *Darb-e Mehr* ("Gate of Mithra") to this day, and when a Zoroastrian priest is initiated he is given a *gurz* (the bull-headed mace of Mithra), as his ritual power is derived from the god.

Dual Gods of Cosmic Order

"O strong Mithra, by an agreement of given promises give us this boon which we ask of you: wealth, strength and victoriousness, well-being and possession of Truth, good reputation and peace of soul, intelligence, increment and knowledge, and Ahura-created Victoriousness, and Best Truth's conquering superiority, and the ability to interpret the Spənta Māthra, so that we being in good spirits, cheerful, joyful, optimistic, may conquer all opponents." Mihr Yašt 10.33

In order to understand Mithra, it is once again necessary to look at him from an Indo-Aryan perspective. Mithra is the equal of Ahura Mazdā because Mitrá is the equal of Varuṇa. In the Vedic tradition, Mitrá and Varuṇa are invoked as a *dvanda* (pair): Mitrāvaruṇa. Their aspects are intrinsically connected, but Mitrá has almost no personal aspects, despite being the first name in the pair. Varuṇa is the greatest god of the ṚgVeda aside from Indra; he is the universal king, and kṣatra (sovereignty) is particularly applicable to him.

The pair of celestial gods are conceived as young and their eye is the sun. They reach out and drive the sun with their arms. Their abode is golden and in the highest heaven. They are kings and universal monarchs. They are called *asuras* (lords) who wield dominion over *māyā* (occult power) and they use this power to send dawns, make the sun traverse the sky, and obscure it with cloud and rain.

They bestow rain on pastures. They are rulers and guardians of the whole world. Their ordinances are fixed and cannot be obstructed by men or gods. They uphold *Ṛta* (Order/Truth) and are barriers against falsehood, which they hate and punish.

"We worship Mithra... who gives neither power nor strength to any man false to a covenant, who gives neither Xvarənah nor reward to any man false to a covenant." Mihr Yašt 10.56

No true understanding of Indo-Iranian religious thought is possible without understanding the key concept of *Aša* (Vedic *Ṛta*, Greek *Kosmos*, Latin *Ratio*): Truth or Cosmic Order. Truth is found in the spring of highest heaven. It is extracted from the waters there (the waters of Chaos). Varuṇa is a water deity: his seat is in the waters. Mitrá, who shares these functions, has his seat in fire. Both are guardians of Truth. In the Vedic material, this is the only major difference that separates the two gods. Otherwise, they are just two sides of the highest heavenly power.

Mitrá is the right hand, Varuṇa is the left. Mitrá embodies the pact between two parties that is tested by fire. Varuṇa personifies the individual oath, tested by water.

Varuna is the terrible "binder." He is the magician who has power over the laws of nature. He is night, sinister, and water.

Mitrá is the contract friend of gift-exchange, pacts, and friendship (contracts and gift-exchange are one and the same in the Indo-European world). He is day, dexter, and fire. His name is connected to the Sanskrit term *mitradrúh* ("covenant breaker" or "friend betrayer"), indicating one who breaks the laws of Mitrá and is worthy of divine punishment.

"Mithra of wide pastures will promote all supreme authorities of the countries and pacify those in revolt."
Fravardīn Yašt 13.95

Mitrá and Varuna are of a class of deities called *Ādityas* in the *Vedas*. *Ādityas* are all concerned with the "contract" as they are gods of the priestly class. The *Āditya* Aryamán ("Aryan-ness") was the personification of social identity, which carried through to Avestan Airyaman who was responsible for marriage rites. The *Āditya* Bhága ("portion") was the apportioner – the divine handout and arbiter of good fortune; he again carried through to Avestan Bagā, which came to be another word for "deity." These other *Ādityas*, including the warlike Indra, faded into minor gods or aspects of Mithra in the Iranian tradition. The Avestan *Aməša Spənta*, who also faded in importance, are similar to the Vedic *Ādityas*.

Varuna's name has the root *vṛ*, meaning to "confine" or "restrict." Originally Varuna was an epithet of the god Asura ("Lord"). Later they were flipped and *Asura* became the title of Varuna.

Asura Varuṇa is "Lord Confining." His Avestan counterpart Ahura Vouruṇā was transformed into Ahura Mazdā: "Lord Wise." Mitrá's name is rooted in the words *mī* ("contract" or "covenant") and *tra* ("tool"). He is the personification of the contract, pact, or alliance. His name also means "friend."

He is the god who regulates the sanctity of agreements between men. He is the guarantor of security and peace. While Vouruṇā changed to Mazdā, he was also absorbed into Avestan Mithra, who rose to prominence in Iranian culture.

"We worship Mithra... who makes the pillars of the high-built house, who makes strong the gateposts." Mihr Yašt 10.28

Mithra came to surpass Ahura Mazdā among the elite. He is called *mazišto yazatō* ("greatest god") in the *Younger Avesta*. Mithra was worshipped throughout the ascendency of Ahura Mazdā. Vouruṇā never recovered his original role or name in the *Avesta*, but Mithra did. Mithra and Ahura are inseparable – they are interdependent. Ahura does not enter into combat (neither do his Vedic and Greek counterparts Varuṇa and Ouranos), instead relying on Mithra to be his active right hand.

Once in Iran, Mithra takes on the military role once occupied by Indra. He ceases to be a magician and becomes god of the warrior contract. This is the oath of the reconstituted honourable *männerbund*, opposed to the lawless band of Indra.

Mithra is no longer associated with the pecuniary debt of the old order, but of the blood oaths and contracts of the warrior elite. Cattle still come under his protection, because any contract or oath requires a physical token of exchange. Cattle were the preferred means of this to the warrior class, leading Mithra the warrior to carry the title *wourugaoyaoiti* ("possessing wide pastureland").

"We worship Mithra of wide cattle pastures with haoma-containing milk and baresman twigs, with skill of tongue and magic word, with speech and action and libations, and with correctly uttered words." Mihr Niyayeš 15

Mithra is "he who calls people to account." Ahura Mazdā remains the left-handed binding god: a priestly lord. Mithra is the right-handed warrior contract god.

Mithra sees men are paid back; that they fulfil their commitments. He punishes those who break their word. He is the warrior who severs the binding with his incorruptible right hand. The right-handed salute of Mithra is the same as that used by the Greeks to Apollon and by the Romans. The right-handed ritual handshake of covenant between men and gods (Greek *dexiosis*, Latin *dextrarum iunctio*) belongs to Mithra also.

Mithra protects the WarYogin as his conduct is in Order. He does not invoke the wrath of Ahurā, who binds those transgressing against ancestral Cosmic Law.

Warrior of Light

"We worship Mithra... the profound, the powerful Lord, granting profit, eloquent, pleased with praise, lofty, very skilful, tanu māthra, the strong-armed warrior." Mihr Yašt 10.25

Ahura Mazdā was frozen in his role, but Mithra's roles expanded. One of the most important was his connection with Light and the sun. Mithra becomes the Light-bringer, herald of Light and Order. He is associated with the sun and Light but is not the actual sun which is personified by the god Hvarəxšaēta.

Mithra is the luminous aether of the heavens, who drives his "one-wheeled golden chariot" (the sun) across the sky, drawn by "supernatural white, radiant, shining, wise, shadowless steeds." He is the light of daybreak and guide of the sun, but not the Dog Star who is personified as another god, Tištrya.

According to the *Mehr Yašt*, a hymn to Mithra, he travels "in front of the sun" and is *hvāroxšna* ("endowed with his own light"). While some scholars have theorised he is the Morning and Evening Star, this is not the case as according to *Mehr Yašt* 10.154 Ahura Mazdā and Mithra are worshipped "as well as the stars, the moon, and the sun." He is not the sun, the moon, or a star: he is a supernatural god.

"We worship Mithra... who is the first supernatural god to approach across the Hara, in front of the immortal swift-horsed

sun; who is the first to seize the beautiful gold-painted mountain-tops; from there the Most Mighty surveys the whole land inhabited by the Aryans." Mihr Yašt 10.12-13

Mithra is born from the waters, and like the sun rises from the waters. These are the waters of the Cosmic Ocean *Vourukaša*. He is "the first to seize the gold-pointed mountain-tops," initially illuminating the Cosmic Mountain *Harā Bərəzaitī*, which is later extrapolated into Roman Mithras being born of a rock.

He brings the sleeping "civilised world" back to life with Light. He is a giver of Light, but only the seed of the "giver of life" exists in the Iranian Mithra. This seed would become the main aspect of the Roman Mithras.

The sun goes behind *Harā Bərəzaitī* at night, but Mithra does not accompany it. He turns back to continue his fight against evil through the hours of darkness. After midnight, Mithra leaves Paradise, located above *Harā Bərəzaitī*, with the god Rašnu on his right.

He arrives east of *Harā Bərəzaitī* at daybreak - the dawn light is due to him. From the east he crosses *Harā Bərəzaitī* on his way west. At sunset he turns around, with Rašnu on his left, and reconnoitres the whole earth. He returns to Paradise before midnight.

"No material man in existence is endowed with greater insight than that which supernatural Mithra is endowed with." Mihr Yašt 10.107

According to both the *Mehr Yašt* and *Vīdēvdāt*, Mithra assists the ascension of the soul as he assists the rising of the sun. He is sleepless, "wakeful in darkness," and "undeceivable." As the never-sleeping watcher of the covenant, he protects and destroys.

Even though he has this route, he is omnipresent and ever watchful. Like Vedic Indra, he has ten thousand unblinking eyes. Despite this association with the nocturnal, no trace of an Underworld element exists in Avestan Mithra.

It is clear that Mithra is not a sun god. He is the god of Light and Order, like Greek Apollon. He later becomes the sun god in the same manner as Apollon does when mixed with other Indo-European gods.

The Parthian word *meh* means "sun," possibly tying their worship of Mithra more specifically to the sun itself. Book 15 of Greco-Roman historian Strabo's *Geography* (63 BCE-24 CE) is the earliest historical reference to Mithra explicitly worshipped as the sun, where he states the Iranians "worship the sun also, whom they call Mithras."

"May you be swift-horsed, like the Sun! May you be resplendent, like the moon! May you be hot-burning, like fire! Mayest you have piercing rays, like Mithra! May you be tall-formed and victorious, like the devout Sraośa!" Āfrīn ī Zartošt 6

Mithra was conflated with Apollon in the syncretic religion of Greek Persia after Alexander, becoming Apollo-Mithra (like Zeus-Ohrmasdes) in the Hellenistic Greco-Zoroastrian Pantheon. To the Armenians and later Iranians he was Mehr. This name for the god still exists in modern Persian as the word for both the sun and "Light" (as in the title of Shah Mohammed Reza Pahlavi: *Aryamehr* – "Light of the Aryans").

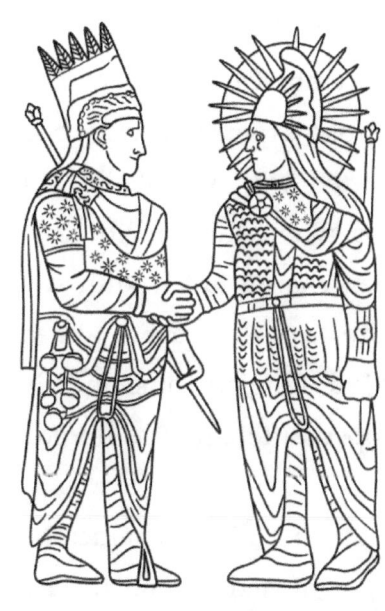

The Armenian king Antiochus I of Commagene built a tomb-sanctuary on Mount Nemrut (now in modern Turkey) in 62 BCE. Large statues of the syncretic Greco-Iranian pantheon were carved, including Apollo-Mithras-Helios-Hermes. The iconography shows the syncretic Mithras – now adorned with a Phrygian cap – with a sunburst behind his head giving the unmistakable right-handed handshake to Antiochus, showing the king's legitimacy.

This development in Armenian territory is the result of Armenia being a buffer between Rome and Parthia. It was the place where the two cultures collided. It marks the point of transition from Iranian Mithra to Hellenic and Roman Mithras, so favoured by the legionaries and soldiers of the Empire.

"We worship Mithra of wide pastures, whose speech is correct, who is eloquent, who has a thousand ears, is well built, has ten thousand eyes, is tall, has a wide outlook, is strong, sleepless, ever-waking, whom rulers descending on the battlefield worship as they advance against blood thirsty enemy armies, against those drawn up in battle lines between the two warring countries." Mihr Yašt 10.7-8

This embrace by the later Roman army is logical, as Mithra's other great role expansion was becoming god of the warrior band. Contrasted with the Vedic Mitrá, Avestan Mithra is a powerful warrior who sallies forth to battle on his spirit-fashioned, star-adorned chariot laden with weapons. He uses his mace to smash oath-breakers. Mithra may already have had the germ of martial traits in the Indo-Iranian homeland. Once the Iranians came to Iran, Mithra developed differently from Vedic Mitrá, who was priestly.

Mithra's military characteristics, as destroyer of oath-breakers, were heightened among the Iranians, who did not elevate Indara (Vedic Indra) like their Indo-Aryan cousins. Once Indara was fully demonised, Mithra came to the fore as god of the ruling warrior caste. Mithra is an enforcer: a punisher of covenant breakers.

This is what led to his adoption by the warrior class, to whom compacts were of the highest importance. Mithra is god of explicit and unspoken contracts both paternal and fraternal. Oaths were sworn over fire: the element of Mithra who is Lord of Fire.

"Such a ruler may be seen above the sun with swift horses."
Dādestān ī Dēnīg 2.14

Mithra is also god of the community social compact – of social structure (caste system). He represents the divine ruler who is of the warrior caste. The warrior class not only worshipped Mithra as *Xšathrapati* ("Lord of Power"), but also saw their leaders as partaking of *Mithraxšathra* ("having rule through Mithra").

As life giver, he is bestower of sons and noble progeny. He is god of the nation's prosperity and welfare. Like Ahura, Mithra remains guardian of *Aša*: Order and Law.

The Iranians extended their moral system onto the battlefield, bringing order to combat where disorder had reigned since the invading cattle raiders of Zarathuštra's time.

Mithra is god of the international treaty, destroying defiant "non-Aryan" nations that do not worship him. In this role he is judge, a characteristic he shares with the legalist Vedic Mitrá. He holds this function implicitly on the battlefield through his companion Rašnu, and explicitly as judge of the dead on the *Činvat Bridge* along with Rašnu and Sraoša.

As judge, Mithra has a thousand eyes and ears. He is ever awake, always watching, nothing escapes his notice – none can outrun him. Spears thrown at him will fly backwards towards his enemies and his mace breaks the skulls of the wicked *daēvas*.

"May Mihr be thy judge, who shall wish thy existence to be vigorous!" Šayest Na-Šayest 22.16

According to the *Mehr Yašt*, Mithra is "the powerful brave warrior" and "strong helper." He is "master of the world," protector and guardian of all creatures. Mithra may have taken on these traits from the *daēvas* Indara and Saurva (Vedic Indra and Śarva/Rudra) when they were demonised, or may simply have had these aspects heightened among the Iranians before the daēvic downfall.

Regardless of the order, Mithra replaces Indara as god of the warband in Iran. He takes on distinctly Indaric qualities in addition to his solar characteristics as "friend" and "contractor."

Mithra is worshipped with libations of *haoma* (a sacrifice he has taken over from Indara), but he does not get drunk on the draught. Mithra is called "replenisher of waters" and "rain-pourer" who "makes plants grow." He frees the waters in the same manner that Indra of the *ṚgVeda* does in the Indic tradition.

"The vices of warriors are oppression, violence, promise-breaking, unmercifulness, ostentation, haughtiness, and arrogance." Dādestān ī Mēnōg ī Xrad 59.8

The Iranian mythos is not later than the Vedic. Both are developments of the Indo-European root that diverged once they arrived in different lands. In India, Indra absorbs Vṛtrahán (slayer of the serpent Vṛtra). This figure is kept separate in Iran becoming Vərəthragna, a member of Mithra's warband. Mithra has the *vazra* (Vedic *vajra*) as his mace, which is Indra's weapon in the Vedic tradition.

Rather than Avestan Indara's traits being divided among other deities, it could have been the Indians who consolidated them in the single god Indra. Vərəthragna, Mithra the mace-wielder, and Thaētaona (slayer of the serpent Dahāka) could have been amalgamated into Indra in the *Vedas*. They may have been separate gods in the original homeland.

"We worship the good, strong, beneficent Fravašis of the righteous, who have metal helmets, metal weapons, metal shields; who fight in battles surrounded by light." Fravardīn Yašt 12.1

The way the divide occurred and the order of events is not important, but the meaning is. The Iranians refined the warband and its leadership, making them take a more moral stance. The host of Indra in Vedic India are the *Maruts* – violent storm gods capable of highly destructive acts. In Iran, the *Fravaši* ancestor spirits have the *Maruts'* role.

The *Fravašis* are unique to Iran, with some characteristics of the Vedic *Pitṛ* (ancestors), as well as embodying the Spirit of the manifold soul. Forming Mithra's retinue, the *Fravašis* are armed and clad in metal armour and drive chariots. Fighting alongside Mithra and his elite command, they are his warriors: his *männerbund*.

Indra is a savage god, and Mithra more refined. Both are gods of the WarYogin. He maintains a fierce and cultured side, using what qualities the situation dictates.

Haoma-drinking Bull Slayer

The spring equinox *Nowruz* festival is balanced by the autumnal equinox by *Mehragān* (Old Persian: *Mithrakāna*). This is the festival of Mithra, which is ancient and deeply embedded in the Indo-Iranian religion.

Mehragān is the only festival where Ahura Mazdā is not invoked as part of the ceremony. It is when, in the mythological record, Thraētaona (Ferēdūn of the epics) slays the serpent king Aži Dahāka (epic Zahhāk) in revenge for the killing of king Yima Xšaēta (epic Jamšid), the primordial ruler who established *Nowruz*, restoring balance to the Cosmos.

The association of Mithra with this festival may appear arbitrary. This is when compared to the winter solstice *Yaldā* festival, which celebrates the culmination of the sun's dying trajectory and the eve of Mithra's Cosmic rebirth.

However, *Mehragān* is symbolic of completion and the end of the current cycle. This is because it is then that which grows reaches perfection: ripeness. It is time to harvest what has reached its end.

The festival originally culminated in the bull sacrifice to Mithra, an act recreating the original bovine sacrifice to bring animal life into the world. This act was primally that of Mithra in the Indo-Iranian religion.

"Hail, bounteous bull! Hail to thee, beneficent bull! Hail to thee, who makest increase! Hail to thee, who makest growth!"
Vīdēvdāt 21.1

It was Zarathuštra and his subsequent adherents who made Aešma (Angra Mainyu) bull slayer, as through their moral lens they considered it an evil act. Originally, Mithra was bull slayer; he was not immoral, since from death comes life and fecundity. This aspect was seized upon by the Roman cult of Mithras, which celebrated the *taurobolium* (bull sacrifice) as a central theme. The sacrifice of a bull on *Mehragān* was sponsored by the rulers of Iran long after the Zarathuštrian reforms frowned upon it. In the *Younger Avesta*, Mithra is averse to blood sacrifices, but that did not stop them being offered to him by kings.

This can be symbolically seen in the reliefs of the lion killing the bull at the palace of Persepolis. The lion is Mithra, the solar totem that slays the lunar bull. It symbolises Hvarəxšaēta (Sun) and Mångha (Moon), summer and winter, warrior and priest. It is emblematic of the cycle of death and rebirth.

In the *Vedas* the moon is the vessel containing the *soma* (Avestan *haoma*) drunk by the gods, specifically Indra. In Iran, this is depicted as Mithra, the lion of the sun eating the bull of the moon.

> *"Up! rise up, thou Moon, that dost keep in thee the seed of the bull."* Vīdēvdāt 21.9

In the Vedic mythos, Mitrá reluctantly participates in the sacrifice of the god Soma, who appears in the shape of a white bull associated with the moon. According to the Avesta, Aŋgra Mainyu kills the primeval bull, whose seed is rescued by Mångha (Moon) as the source for all other animals. In the Roman myth, Mithras – associated with the unconquered sun – must slay the bull of the moon each month in order for life to be regenerated.

The original Indo-Iranian myth can be reconstituted from these traditions. Mithra, solar god of light, kills the life-giving Cosmic bull so its blood and semen (the *haoma* draught) fertilises all vegetation and animals. This is the ritualistic prototype of fertility in the Indo-Iranian Mithraic cult of the *Karapan* priests the Avesta denounces.

> *"Even the slightest pressing of Haoma, even the slightest praise of Haoma, even the slightest drink of Haoma serves to slay a thousand daēvas."* Hōm Yašt, Yasna 10.6

Haoma (literally "The thing which has been pressed") refers to the juice of a plant personified in a god called Haoma (Pahlavi: Hōm). The identity of *haoma* is unknown, but could have been the ephedra plant, which fits the description of the plant and effects of consuming it.

The real *haoma* only existed in the original homeland. Substitutes that did not have the properties of the original were used by Iranian and Indic people, who no longer had access to it.

The *asu* (stalks) of *haoma* yielded a yellow juice called "yellow *haoma*." It grew in the mountains, and the *Hōm Yašt* says the god Haoma was deposited on *Harā Bərəzaitī*. Birds then carried him to other mountain peaks.

Once pressed, the juice *haoma* was also the god Haoma. It was always a manifestation of the god, infused with divine personality and sacred power. *Haoma* was intoxicating but did not make one drunk. *Yašt* 10.8 states "that intoxication which is Hōm's is accompanied by gladdening Truth."

"I am Haoma the true death dispeller." Hōm Yašt, Yasna 9.1.3

It was a stimulant taken before battle, enhancing mental capabilities and perception. *Haoma* allowed the drinker to grasp Truth. In the *Avesta*, the *haoma*-drinker collapses the boundaries between the worlds; he erases the distinction between himself and the divine.

Haoma is drunk during ritual, but also before battle. Heroes are the primary practitioners of the cult of Haoma, who is invoked for victory on the battlefield. Mithra drinks *haoma* before going into battle.

This is ritualised through the central Indo-Iranian *haoma* sacrifice still central to Zoroastrian ritual. There it is poured into the emblematic fire of Mithra.

Haoma blesses those who brew him with virility, but belongs only to the righteous. He curses with sterility those who fail to honour him. In *Yasna* 9, Haoma assists the propagation of the heroic generation.

The seed of the hero who has drunk *haoma* gains strength. The fiery seed of the father gives a blazing *Xvarənah* ("light of glory") to the son. The first four men said to have pressed *haoma* each received the boon of a great son: Vivanghvant who had Yima, Athwya who had Thraētaona, Thrita who had Kərśaspa, and Pouruśaspa who had Zarathuśtra.

"Haoma allots power and strength to heroes." Hōm Yašt, Yasna 9.22

Thrita was the third man who prepared *haoma* for the corporeal world. He appears under two names: Thrita the healer and preparer of *haoma*, and Thraētaona (Feridun in epic) who slays the three-headed serpent Aži Dahāka in the early iteration of the dragonslayer myth.

In later mythos, Thraētaona (who represents the pastoral caste) clubs Aži Dahāka about the head, neck, and heart. However he cannot slay him, instead imprisoning the wounded monster under Mount Damāvand.

His son Kərəsāspa (representing the warrior caste), who slays the sea monster Gaṇdarəwa, will be resurrected to finish the work of Thraētaona by defeating Aži Dahāka in the final battle of the Cosmic cycle. Haoma is also critical to the warriors of this battle. The "*White Haoma*" (also called *Gaokarena*), which grows on *Hūkairya* (one of the celestial peaks), will help the Army of Light defeat the forces of Darkness.

The dragon slaying myth is intrinsically tied to *haoma* lore, as evidenced in the Vedic material, where the serpent Vṛtra is transformed into the god Soma, the lunar bull. In the *Younger Avesta* the primordial man Gayō Marətan is substituted for the first king Yima who is sacrificed by the wicked Aži Dahāka, setting off the chain of events that culminate in the defeat of the serpent by *haoma*-sacrificing Thraētaona. The slaying of Yima is marked by *Nowruz*, the defeat of Aži Dahāka is celebrated on *Mehragān*, where the lunar bull of *haoma* is sacrificed to Mithra marking the cycle's completion.

"I call down, O yellow Haoma, your intoxicating power, strength, victoriousness, health, curativeness, prosperity, growth, force for the entire body, complete knowledge, I call down this that I may go about among beings autonomously, overcoming hostility, defeating the Lie." Hōm Yašt, Yasna 9.17

The Pahlavi *Rivāyat* book states that the left eye of the animal is offered to Haoma during the sacrifice as the first portion. The left eye is the moon; the right eye is the sun.

The first offering of the bull of *haoma* is offered to Haoma, giving strength to the god so he can in turn give strength to Mithra. This aspect of the Mithraic cult is preserved by the Kurdish Yazidis ("Deity worshippers") and Ahl-e Haqq ("People of the Truth"), both of whom still preserve the myth of the primordial contract sealed by the sacrifice of a bull.

The WarYogin drinks the *haoma* and swears a powerful oath to Mithra over his internal fire, making a covenant with his Self. He sees Mithra present wherever the Cosmic power of deliverance is present: in the victory of life over death, Light over Darkness, sunrise, the release of the waters in spring. He understands the rising sun manifests Mithra's victorious power over the forces of the netherworld both without and within.

"I invoke Mithra, the lord of the wide pastures, a god armed with beautiful weapons, with the most glorious of all weapons, with the most victorious of all weapons." Vīdēvdāt 19.15

Mithra is the Celestial WarYogin; he provides the model for the WarYogin to emulate. He is the holy warrior of Light who fights against the forces of Darkness with an incorruptible right hand. He fights for Order and Truth, smashing the agents of chaos and those who break their word, joining the powers of dissolution.

Mithra is ever vigilant; he is always watching and manning the ramparts ready for enemy attack. Mithra has absolute supremacy in insight and physical prowess. He is mightiest, strongest, most mobile, fastest, and most victorious.

Mithra is both fair and forgiving, but carries out his militant justice with his own hand, not devolving the role to another. He is a mediator who arbitrates the contract defining terms of engagement between Ohrmazd and Ahriman during the Cosmic war. As the Contract, Mithra is the link connecting upper and lower worlds. He is mediator between the Cosmic poles, realising Totality by balancing antagonistic forces.

The WarYogin invokes Mithra, *Xvarənah*, and the *Fravaṣis* before going into battle within himself.

"[Mithra] who sets the battle in motion, who takes his stand in battle, who, taking his stand in battle, smashes the battle lines." Mihr Yašt 10.36

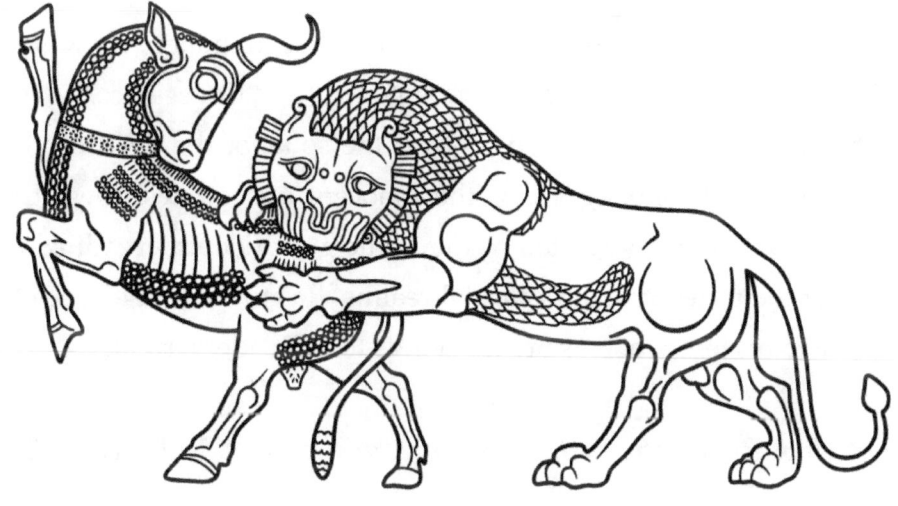

Mithra's Warband

"I invoke the mighty Fravaşis of the righteous. I invoke Vərəthragna, made by Ahurā, who wears the Glory made by Mazda. I invoke Tištrya, the bright and glorious star, in the shape of a golden-horned bull." Vīdēvdāt 19.37

Mithra is god of the warband: a group of sworn brothers pledged to fraternal alliance through covenant and friendship. As lord of the warrior loyalty oath, Mithra is accompanied by his own powerful band of warriors. His large retinue is comprised of powerful deities including Sraoša, Rašnu, Vərəthragna, Vayu, Ātar, *Xvarənah*, Aši, and the *Fravaşis*.

Accompanying Mithra on either side as his attendants are Rašnu ("Justice") and Sraoša ("Obedience," "Conscience," or "Observance"), his fellow judges over the souls of the dead on the *Činvat Bridge*. Rašnu fights for the innocent and strikes down the guilty. He is possibly related to the Vedic god Viṣṇu, pervading all parts of the terrestrial and celestial realms. Rašnu the Judge attends Mithra to his left, whereas Sraoša stands to his leader's right.

"Then Rašnu the tall, the strong, will come." Rašn Yašt 12.6

Ahura Mazdā created Sraoša to fight against the demon of wrath, Aēšma (who is later known as Aṅgra Mainyu). He was first to offer prayer and chant the *Gāthās*. He keeps armed sleepless vigil over the entire Cosmos, day and night. After the sun sets, he drives the demons back into the Darkness. Sraoša (later called Sorūsh) is the spirit of wakefulness. Embodied by the sacred rooster Parōdarš, he counteracts the efforts of the demoness Būšyanstā ("Futurity") who sabotages the daily progress of men causing them to adopt the attitude of "what will be will be."

Mithra chases the armies "hither," Rašnu chases them "thither," and Sraoša scatters them. Aši ("Reward") is a constant companion of Sraoša and chariot driver of Mithra; she is goddess of fortune and the moral advocate and compass for women. Ātar ("Fire") is another of Mithra's close companions, lighting the straight path of Truth. In front of the retinue flies *Xvarənah*, nimbus of glory. The fiery *Xvarənah* ("Glory" or "Fortune") embodies both semen and the blazing halo of legitimate rule: sign of a divine king.

"The holy Sraoša, the best protector of the poor, is fiend-smiting; he is the best smiter of the Lie." Sroš Yašt Hādōxt 11.3

Vərəthragna

"Then strongest Vərəthragna said to him: In strength I am the strongest, in valour the most valorous, in Xvarənah I am the most in possession of Xvarənah." Wahrām Yašt 14.3

Mithra the Enforcer is also assisted by Vərəthragna ("Obstruction Smiter"), god of victory. Vərəthragna slays enemies in battle and brings disease and death to those who deceive Mithra. He is the Iranian reflection of Indra as dragonslayer (Vedic Vṛtrahán – "Destroyer of Vṛtra").

Indra as dragonslayer may stem from the Indo-Iranian/Indo-Aryan god *Vrtraghna. However the actual act of killing Aži Dahāka, also known as Vərəthra (Vedic Vṛtra), is done by the culture hero Thraētaona. His son Kərəsāspa – another central Avestan culture hero – is also a dragonslayer, killing Aži Sruvara.

Vərəthragna (later called Bahrām or Wahrām) is god of combat. He is the best-armed of all gods. He conquers demons; he is the wild boar and bestower of the *Xvarənah*.

Vərəthragna epitomises the ideal of an "*Aryan* warrior." Fiercely aggressive, smashing the defences of all who stand in his way, he expresses the aggressive, irresistible force of victory through offensive warfare. He is accompanied by the goddess Vanaintī Uparatāt ("Conquering Superiority").

"Ahura-created Vərəthragna came driving to him a fifth time in the form of a ferocious wild boar with sharp teeth, with sharp tusks, a boar that kills at one blow, unapproachable when angered, prepared for battle, outflanking the enemy." Wahrām Yašt 14.15

Vərəthragna has ten incarnations, each of which expresses a dynamic force of the god. The first avatar is the strong wind Vāta Vərəthrajan ("Victorious Wind"), who is also a god in his own right named Vayu. The second is a powerful bull with yellow ears and golden horns. Third is a white horse with golden ears and a golden bridle. Fourth is a burden-bearing, sharp-toothed, rutting camel who stamps his way forward. His fifth form, his most prominent, is that of a boar. The sharp-tusked male boar kills with one stroke; he is wrathful and strong, clearing the way for Mithra. Sixth is that of a handsome youth of fifteen.

The seventh form of Vərəthragna, a falcon, is also significant. Vərəthragna is closely associated with *Xvarənah*, which he carries like a battle standard bestowing upon the victor. *Xvarənah* fled the first king Yima when he fell from grace in the form of a falcon, going to Mithra, Thaētaona, and Kərəsāspa. Vərəthragna's bird form is also associated with the raven. The ancient Persians viewed a raven's feathers with superstitious awe as they were thought to make a man inviolable, bringing him prosperity as well as glory.

"Ahura-created Vərəthragna came driving to him a seventh time in the form of a falcon, seizing from below with its talons, crushing from above with its beak, who is the fastest of birds, the swiftest of those that fly forth." Wahrām Yašt 14.19

Vərəthragna's eighth form is a wild ram, ninth a fighting buck goat, and tenth a warrior holding a sword with a golden blade. All of his avatars are aggressive and virile. In later Greek-Iranian syncretism, Vərəthragna is conflated with Herakles.

In the late Achaemenid period, a custom began of carrying embers from a sacred fire before the Persian army as it advanced. This Ātar-Vərəthragan ("Victorious Fire" or "Fire of Wahrām") acted as an emblem of victory, a palladium for the Iranian warriors going into battle.

Vayu

"My name is Vayu, O holy Zarathuštra! My name is Vayu, because I go through the two worlds, the one which the Good Spirit has made and the one which the Evil Spirit has made." Rām Yašt 15.43

The wind god Vayu is associated with the warrior band in both Avestan and Vedic cultures. Vedic Vāyú becomes more prominent in Iran as Vayu, god of the *männerbund* and warrior society. His name means "Wind," one of the key elements (along with fire) of the hero.

Vayu is a skilful fighter. It is the swift nature of the god tying him to the youthful warrior. Vayu is first to receive sacrifice among the war gods, stating his importance to war. The *Rām Yašt* says he "wears the raiment of warfare."

Vayu straddles the material realm and Otherworld. He traverses and fills the void between opposites. This is a trait the young wolf warrior aims to emulate.

Vayu may have been above Indara in an earlier strata of Indo-Iranian/Indo-Aryan religion. Indra's ascendency over Vāyú is likely to be a Vedic development. In the *Vedas*, Indra had Vāyú as a regular companion.

Vāyú was brutal and furious. Indra had beauty and dexterity. In Iran, Indra became the demon Indara, while Vayu lost some of his brutal edge, yet remained a fierce warrior.

Armed with a club, the fierce hero Kərəsāspa is connected to the cult of Vayu. His father Thraētaona does not display Vayu-like characteristics. This is because he is connected to the cattleman caste, whereas Kərəsāspa is definitively a member of the warrior caste.

"Vayu, swift, high-girdled, possessing from yoke-thongs, high-stepping, broad-chested, broad-hipped." Rām Yašt 15.54

Vayu is invoked in time of peril. When proper sacrifice is made to him, he averts danger and teaches men magic spells to fight demons. In the *Avesta*, both Ahura Mazdā and Aŋgra Mainyu offer sacrifice to Vayu.

Vayu is an ambiguous god with traits of both Light and Dark – he has the air of neutrality about him. Vayu straddles the line between *daēva* and good *yazata*.

In his dark aspect of destroyer, he severs the soul from the body. In his light aspect as guide, he transports the souls of the dead to the *Činvat Bridge* where they are judged by Mithra.

The Avesta differentiates between two different wind gods: Vayu and Vāta. Vāta is the physical wind, particularly associated with Mithra and Vərəthragna; the elemental force. Vayu is always a distinct personality from the physical wind: the metaphysical Wind. While Vayu is always the name of the god, *vāta* can also be used to simply mean "wind."

Asman (stone vault of heaven) is separated from the earth by void. This void is where Vāta and Vayu operate. Later *Pahlavi* literature takes these two gods and conflates them with the two sides of Vayu, calling them *vāy ī veh* (good wind) and *vāy ī badtar* (evil wind).

"Then I shall overcome hostilities, the hostilities of all enemies, the hostilities of daēvas and men, sorcerers and witches, tyrants, Kavis and Karapans." Wahrām Yašt 14.4

While Avestan Vayu is complex with both destroyer and resurrector characteristics, he is still a moral force compared with his Vedic counterpart. He, like all members of the Iranian war host, always fights on the side of Light and *Aša*.

The Iranian gods mark a moment of rehabilitation and refinement of the Indo-European *männerbund*. The wolf warriors become "Noble Wolves," and the warrior evolves beyond hunter and raider. He becomes the heroic protector, defender, and conqueror.

The WarYogin is the Noble Wolf. He embodies the heroic ideals of duty, self-sacrifice and honour, while not allowing his teeth to become dull. He stays violent like Vərəthragna and Vayu, smashing through the obstacles that stand in the way of his transcendence, always fighting on the side of Order and Light.

"And Riches will cleave unto him, giving him full welfare, holding a shield before him, powerful, rich of cattle and garments; and Victory will cleave unto him, day after day; and likewise Strength, that smites more than a year. Attended by that Victory, he will conquer the havocking hordes; attended by that Victory, he will conquer all those who hate him. For its brightness and glory, I will offer it a sacrifice..." Zamyad Yašt 8.54

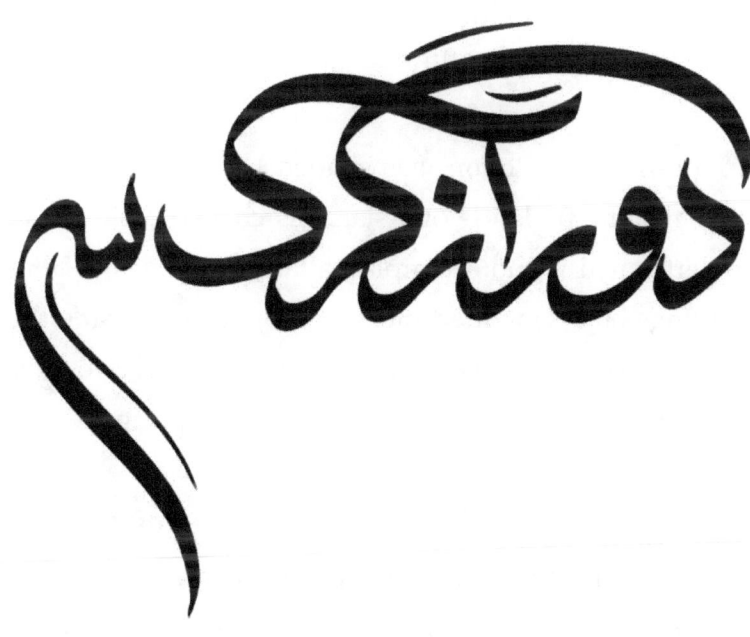

Fire and Water

"All coming to being, maturing, and organising in this world proceeds from a balanced union of the female water and the male fire." Dēnkard 3.80

The connection between Mithra and fire is well established. Water traditionally belongs to Vourunā-Ahura. This is a function that does not pass to Ahura Mazdā, but the third god in the Avestan ahuric triad alongside Mazdā and Mithra: Apąm Napāt. This god is later displaced by water goddess Arədvī Sūrā Anāhitā, who gains popularity among Iran's nobility.

The Indo-Iranian religion was shaped by countless generations wandering the steppe lands of Asia. This created a simple form of worship performed without temples, altars, or statues. Deities were given offerings on a sanctified piece of ground. Alongside the main deities, fire and water received sacrifice. These two could be represented by the domestic fire and household spring.

"Thus, in all areas of philosophy, cosmology, ritual, and mythology, water and fire are always closely and positively related." Philippe Gignoux, Man and Cosmos in Ancient Iran

The connection between fire and water is strong in Avestan philosophy and ritual. Modern Zoroastrianism still maintains the *āb-zōhr* libation rite. This follows the *ātaš-zōhr* fire oblation during the *yasna* ceremony.

These two rituals are always paired and have been since Iranian pre-history. According to eminent Iranologist Mary Boyce, the *Yasna Haptanhāiti* section of the *Avesta* dates back to a pre-Zoroastrian liturgy accompanying the priest's offerings to fire and water. The two rituals are bound together, jointly honouring Mithra and Apąm/Anāhitā.

Fire

"The Fire looks at the hands of all passers-by – 'what does the friend bring to the friend, the one that goes forth to the one that sits still?' We sacrifice unto the holy Fire, the bold, good warrior." Ataš Niyayeš 14

While permanent ever-burning fire temples were not established until the Parthian and Sassanid periods, worship of fire and through fire as an intermediary is part of the deepest layer of the Indo-European religion. Like Haoma, Ātar ("Fire") is an element and a deity; more properly, *ātarš* (physical fire) is a manifestation of Ātar (the god Fire).

Ātar (like Vedic Agni) is an intermediary between men and gods. The *Bundahišn* (18.1-7) relates five manifestations of Ātar: *Bərəzisavah* (transcendent fire which blazes in the presence of Ohrmazd), *Vohufryāna* (which is in the bodies of men and animals), *Urvāzišta* (in plants), *Vāzišta* (in the clouds), and *Spəništa* (that which is kept for work in the material world: mundane fire).

"He fashioned five kinds of fire: the Burzišvang fire, the Hufryān fire, the Urvāzišt fire, the Vāzišt fire, and the Speništ fire." Bundahišn 18.1

In the Iranian tradition, Fire is more than the mouth of the gods, as he is in the Vedic branch. Ātar is the transcendent channel of communication occupying all the levels of existence from the material plane to the throne of the divine. Fire is capable of manifesting in manifold form – it is found in all forms of life.

Light is the original substance of creation. Ohrmazd created the Cosmos from his own *xwadīh* (selfhood/essence). The *xwadīh* of Ohrmazd is *rōšnīh* (Light), while the *xwadīh* of Ahriman is *tārīgīh* (Darkness).

From his formless *asar-rōšnīh* ("Realm of Light"), he created and spread fire as the vivifying element that exists in all levels of the cosmos, both *gētīg* (material) and *mēnōg* (formless). Fire was thus created of and separated from aether, much like in the work of Pre-Socratic Greek philosophers Heraklitos and Anaxagoras. Due to its separation from aether, fire has properties of both Light and air.

Fire is the final of the seven creations of Ohrmazd, but is accorded a special status which setting it apart from the other six (sky, water, earth, plant, cow, and man). The *Bundahišn* 1a.5 relates that Ohrmazd "created the fire ember and joined it to the radiance of the endless Light." Fire connects the lowest to the highest planes of existence.

"And in the beginning of the creation the whole earth was delivered over into the guardianship of the sublime Farrobāg fire, the mighty Gušnasp fire, and the beneficial Burzēnmihr fire, which are like priest, warrior, and husbandman."
Vizīdagīhā ī Zādspram 11.8

Three supreme sacred fires burned in pre-Islamic Iran. Each had its own location, which later had temples built to house them. These fires were said to protect the Iranian homeland from evil. Each represented one of the Indo-Iranian castes and was started by a different mythical Iranian king.

Farrobāg Fire was said to be ignited by Jam (Yima). It represented priestly fire. *Gušnasp* was started by Kay Husrow, the "stallion of the *Aryan* lands." This was the warrior's fire. *Burzēnmihr*, the fire of king Vištāspa, was the farmer's fire.

Ātar is in the retinue of Mithra; because Mithra is the Lord of Fire, he has dominion over the flames. An oath to Mithra, the warrior contract, is made over a sacred fire. Ātar is called on as the bold, good warrior in the *Avesta*. Manifested as Ātar-Vərəthragan, he is required in order to battle the demons of Darkness. This fire, the Fire of Vahrām is the highest form of sacred fire to the warrior.

> *"The Burzišvang fire is the fire burning before Lord Ohrmazd."* Bundahišn 18.2

Fire is the virile, masculine element that burns away Darkness and refines the crude parts of the WarYogin. It tempers and hardens him, stripping away the non-essentials, leaving just the essence. It is his bare Nature that undergoes the purification of water, the alchemical *ablutio* that washes away impurities.

The water allows the WarYogin's Spirit to regain its original purity and travel on the path of fire. Fire is the route the WarYogin follows, connecting the fire in his original Essence to that which burns in the presence of Ohrmazd. He returns this fire to its source, attaining his incorruptible *tan ī pasēn* ("final body"): his original luminous body of light.

Burning Water

> *"All the shores around the Sea Vourukaša are in commotion, the whole middle is bubbling up."* Ābān Niyayeš 5

In the earliest layers of Avestan religion lies the water deity Apąm Napāt ("Child of the Waters"). This third member of the ahuric trinity has a Vedic counterpart, Apāṃ Napāt, who embodies fire that burns in water. This is an epithet of Vedic fire god Agni, "born from the waters." Iranian scholar Abolala Soudavar has reconstructed Avestan Apąm Napāt's name to have originally meant "Burning Water," stating it was changed on purpose to diminish a once great god.

Mithra's original counterpart Vourunā split in two, with his titles taking on a life of their own as separate gods Apąm Napāt and Ahura Mazdā. This explains why the two Vedic gods Mitrá and Varuṇa become the trinity of Avestan gods (Ahura Mazdā, Mithra, and Apąm Napāt are the only gods with the title *ahura*). Apąm Napāt may have been the original creator god in the Iranian branch until he was supplanted by Ahura Mazdā. His Vedic counterpart Apāṃ Napāt was the one "who has created all beings through his power as *asura*" (*Ṛg Veda* 2.35.2).

"The daēva par excellence was thus Apąm Napāt, the Burning Water who gave life, and was perceived as the main competitor to Ahura Mazdā." Abolala Soudavar, Discrediting Ahura Mazdā's Rival

Apąm Napāt is a fire or brightness in the waters, directly corresponding to the Vedic Apāṃ Napāt. As Abolala Soudavar puts it in his work *Discrediting Ahura Mazdā's Rival*: "There was, however, one god, Apąm Napāt, who presented a serious problem for the *Avesta* compilers. He was a mighty god, an aquatic deity to whom life, and therefore creation, was originally attributed."

Therefore, his creator function was stripped of him, leaving a bare trace of him in the Avestan record.

Mary Boyce also points to this same original function in the *Encyclopaedia Iranica*: "*Yašt* 19.52 shows that in one of his aspects the ancient Apąm Napāt was a mighty creator-god 'who created men, who shaped men'... but in Zoroastrianism Ahura Mazdā is venerated as supreme Creator, and Apąm Napāt thus came to be robbed of this function."

Apąm Napāt's cult title and ancient invocation *Ahura Bərəzant* ("High Lord") was abbreviated to *Ahura*. This over the course of time lead to the transfer of praises originally addressed to him to Ahura Mazdā, the *Ahura* of Zarathuštra.

"The high, lofty, Ahura, having great powers and dominion over the worlds, brilliant, grandchild of the waters, he who has swift horses, we praise. The virile one, who gives help when called upon, he who created heroic men and women, he who fashioned heroic men and women, the hallowed god being amid the waters, who being prayed to is swiftest of all to hear." Zamyād Yašt 19.52

These praises are explicitly devoted to Ahura Mazdā in the Zoroastrian liturgy, but there are clues contained within them that point to a different *ahura*. In *Yasna* 38, the regenerative Waters are called *ahurānīš ahurahyā* ("*ahura's* wives"), making Apąm Napāt the more likely husband than Ahura Mazdā (who is explicitly named in the passage). In *ṚgVeda* 2.32.8 and 7.34.22, the Waters are called *varuṇānī* ("wives of Varuṇa").

To the Medes, Mithra and Apąm Napāt were the complimentary pair: Mithra was a solar god who presided over daytime, while Apąm Napāt was an aquatic god who presided over night-time. This is almost identical to the function of Vedic Mitrá and Varuṇa. The Vedic title Apāṃ Napāt is normally given to Agni the god of fire, but Apāṃ Napāt may have originally been the title of Varuṇa, who is sometimes also Agni.

In Ṛg Veda 10.8.5 the poet, addresses Agni: "You become the eye and protector of great Ṛta (Avestan Aša) – you become Varuṇa, since you enter on behalf of Ṛta, you become Apāṃ Napāt."

"O Waters, now we worship you, you that are showered down, and you that stand in pools and vats, and you that bear forth. Ye female ahuras of Ahura, you that serve us in helpful ways, well forded and full-flowing, and effective for the bathings, we will seek you and for both the worlds!" Yasna 38.3

The connection of Indo-Iranian Apąm Napāt to Vourunā is strengthened by the dwelling place of the *ahura*: the Cosmic Ocean *Vourukaša*, which is etymologically linked with Vourunā. In *Yušt* 19.52, Apąm Napāt is said to have created and formed mankind. He is therefore a principle of life, much like the fire created by Ahura Mazdā in the standard orthodoxy.

So is the *Xvarənah*, a fiery emanation of glory from the celestial Light, which abides with Apąm Napāt in *Vourukaša*. In an interesting Germanic parallel, the ninth century CE Norwegian poet Thjódólf of Hvinir, uses the phrase *sævar niþr* ("grandson/descendant of the sea") as a kenning for fire in his skaldic poem *Ynglingatal*.

The last attested worship of Apąm Napāt was by Achaemenid ruler Artaxerxes III, in the late fourth century BCE. They invoked him alongside Ahura Mazdā and Mithra by another of his cult-names: Baga ("Dispenser"). Baga implies the dispenser of good.

Apąm Napāt is called Baga in the *Avesta* when placed with Mithra. Mithra-Baga is the Indo-Iranian equivalent of Indo-Aryan *dvanda* Mitrāvaruṇa. As Baga, Apąm Napāt sets Haoma on the Cosmic Mountain.

"Swift and wise hath the well-skilled Baga created thee; swift and wise on high Haraitī did He, the well-skilled, plant thee (Haoma)." Yasna 10.10

Anāhita

"From this river of mine alone flow all the waters." Ābān Yašt 5.5

Artaxerxes II (404-359 BCE) displaced Apąm Napāt with Anāhitā, with the goddess replacing the third *ahura* on all of his inscriptions. This was the natural conclusion of his predecessors' devotion to the goddess Arədvī Sūrā Anāhitā, a stellar goddess and water divinity.

Apąm Napāt was made subordinate to the goddess by being turned into the child of Anāhita. The pair are then depicted as mother and infant son.

Some scholars have tried to conflate Anāhitā with the Mesopotamian goddess Ishtar, asserting that pre-Iranian religions of agricultural societies on the Iranian plateau were goddess and fertility based. That in turn, the Indo-European Iranians incorporated some of these goddesses into their warlike male pantheon. While Anāhitā may have later been associated with Ishtar in the syncretic religions of the Hellenistic period and beyond, she was a goddess that the Indo-Iranians brought with them, rather than a local deity.

"All the shores around the Sea Vourukaša are in commotion, the whole middle is bubbling up when she flows forth to them, when she streams forth to them, Arədvī Sūrā Anāhitā." Abān Niyayeš 5

Arədvī Sūrā Anāhitā ("Moist Powerful Unbound") is the Virgin of the Waters, not an Earth Mother. Darius II (423 BCE-404 BCE) officially sanctioned the cult of Arədvī Sūrā Anāhitā the Celestial River goddess that feeds all rivers. Invoked more concisely as Anāhitā, this goddess who accompanies Mithra in later Iranian religion is the embodiment of the Celestial River.

Arədvī Sūrā Anāhitā is an epithet for a goddess named Haraxvatī (Vedic Sárasvatī, Greek Arachōsíā), the river goddess of a forgotten region in the original homeland. Haraxvatī is the Celestial River: the Milky Way. The River of the Celestial Mountain *Harā Bərəzaitī*.

The goddess, whose real name may simply be Āp ("Water"), is described as a "beautiful maiden," who accompanies the boatman Pāurva (Vafra Navaza) to the ground in the Ābān Yašt after he is thrown into the sky by Thraētaona. This is an ecstatic journey, with Paurva another name for *haoma* and the hero Thraētaona (as a bird) as the agent of the magical flight.

Only after invoking Anāhita does the aerial adventure of Paurva come to a close. This connects Anāhita with the *daēnā*, the female celestial double or spirit guide.

"The old Vafra Navaza worshipped her when the strong fiend-smiter, Thraētaona, flung him up in the air in the shape of a bird, of a vulture. He went on flying, for three days and three nights, towards his own house; but he could not, he could not turn down. At the end of the third night, when the beneficent dawn came dawning up, then he prayed unto Arədvī Sūrā Anāhita… Arədvī Sūrā Anāhita hastened unto him in the shape of a maid, fair of body, most strong, tall-formed, high-girdled, pure, nobly born of a glorious race." Ābān Yašt 5.61-64

Anāhita is the only deity to be worshipped in images. Other gods' cults did not use idols, as the Iranians generally did not portray their deities as humans or animals. They remained conceptual, something that continued in the Islamic tradition.

Iranians communed with their gods beyond the human level. The late idolic depictions of the goddess are influenced by the Semitic goddess Ishtar, but Anāhita is an earlier Indo-European goddess with imagery that suggests a far Northern origin.

Worshipped "with the *haoma* and meat," the Northern goddess wears a coat of beaver pelts in the *Ābān Yašt*. Beavers live in the cold climates of the North, not the Near East. Fur is worn in the cold North. This places her in the earlier Indo-Iranian pantheon.

In *Vīdēvdāt* 14, the killing of a "water dog" (beaver) is a high crime with a harsh punishment. Again this reinforces a more ancient and Northerly origin of the goddess and people who worshipped her.

Anāhitā is seen as a waterfall flowing from *Hūkairya*, a high peak of *Harā Bərəzaitī*, the Celestial Mountain connecting sky and earth. This indicates snow melt that flows down mountains in spring. The Northern divinity also drives a chariot pulled by four pure white horses: wind, rain, cloud, and sleet.

"She is clothed with garments of beaver, Arədvī Sūrā Anāhitā; with the skin of thirty beavers of those that bear four young ones, that are the finest kind of beavers; for the skin of the beaver that lives in water is the finest-coloured of all skins, and when worked at the right time it shines to the eye with full sheen of silver and gold." Ābān Yašt 5.129

Anāhitā is the fair maiden: strong, beautiful, high-girt, and straight, shod with gleaming golden shoes. She presides over generation and birth and furthers creatures, the land, the herd, and wealth. Because she is linked with giving life, warriors such as Thraētaona and Kərəsāspa pray to her before battle for victory.

She is described as strong and bright, tall and beautiful, pure and nobly born. As befits her noble birth she wears a golden crown with eight rays and a hundred stars, a golden mantle, and a golden necklace around her beautiful neck.

Anāhitā is associated closely with another goddess: Aši, the chariot driver of Mithra and goddess of fortune. Aši bestows wisdom and guards chastity. She is a noble maiden. Invincible in battle, she grants victory.

Aši possesses healing for waters, animals, and plants, and overcomes both demonic and human enmity. Anāhitā has no moral function, whereas Aši is moral. A strong advocate of female morality, she laments abortion and infidelity.

"We sacrifice to Aši Vanguhī, who is shining, high, tall-formed, well worthy of sacrifice, with a loud-sounding chariot, strong, welfare-giving, healing, with fulness of intellect, and powerful." Aši Yašt 17.1

The two goddesses are intertwined. Water is symbolic of health and healing, functions of both goddesses.

Anāhitā is the indomitable feminine aspect of the dual goddess. Aši is the female principle subordinated to the male principle.

Anāhitā is like untouchable Greek Artemis. Aši is like Athena, the powerful virgin daughter of the father.

Ātar is fire and Apąm Napāt is the fire in water. Mithra is the male principle of fire and Aši-Anāhitā is the female principle of water. Mithra and the goddess (Aši-Anāhitā) are the Iranian reflection of the Indic Śiva and Śakti.

The WarYogin takes these two divine principles and reunites them in his being. He unifies the god and goddess so that he is capable of fighting the Final Battle and attaining total victory on the Cosmic battlefield. Water is the feminine element that purifies the WarYogin after fire has tempered and hardened him to his reduced, essential nature. His fiery essence is quenched in the Celestial River, creating an adamantine edge capable of cutting through the hordes of Darkness and reaching beyond the peak of the Cosmic Mountain.

Light of Glory

"Their body is the fire of the material world, but their soul is Glory coming from the divinities that settle in them." Bundahišn 18.12

Fire is born of Light, yet nurtured in water. Mithra is born of Ohrmazd, or sometimes of Anāhitā in later myths. Ohrmazd, like Vedic Váruṇa is the celestial "chaotic" Waters; Anāhitā is the Celestial River.

Whether born of the Light of Ohrmazd or of Anāhitā, Mithra is born of the Waters of Chaos. This is the realm of non-dual possibilities.

The extraction of fire from water represents Truth extracted from Chaos. Apąm Napāt (the fire in water) represents this also.

One of Apąm Napāt's key functions in the *Avesta* is to protect the *Xvarənah* ("Light of Glory") in the *Vourukaša* ocean when it is in danger of falling into the wrong hands. *Xvarənah* is deified "Glory." The god *Xvarənah* is cognate to Vedic Svarṇara ("Lord of Bright Space" or "Lord of Ether").

The concept *Xvarənah* is equivalent to Greek *dóxa* ("glory") and *tykhe* ("destiny"). *Xvarənah* is a fiery, life-giving emanation of the outer light who dwells in the waters of *Vourukaša*.

"That Glory swells up and goes to the sea Vourukaša. The swift-horsed Son of the Waters seizes it at once: this is the wish of the Son of the Waters, the swift-horsed: 'I want to seize that Glory that cannot be forcibly seized, down to the bottom of the sea Vourukaša, in the bottom of the deep rivers.'" Zamyād Yašt 19.51

Xvarənah is the all-luminous substance – the pure luminescence of which all of Ohrmazd's creatures are constituted at their origin. He is the Energy of sacral Light ensuring victory for the Forces of Light over the demonic Powers of Darkness.

Xvarənah caused Yima to prosper until the monarch's sin caused *Xvarənah* to depart from him in the shape of a falcon. He is protector of the "Aryan lands," of animals, of righteous men, and of the Mazdean religion.

Xvarənah is not an abstract concept. It is a real, physical, though invisible force – the creative power of the gods. It is the privilege of the luminous warriors, priests, and cattlemen of the *Arya*.

After Apąm Napāt seized the *Xvarənah*, Ahura Mazdā made the attainment of it a legitimate goal of striving by qualified humans, granting sacerdotal, pastoral, and martial rewards. *Xvarənah* has solar origins. Like the sun, it triumphs over Darkness.

It is the supernatural fire, the dazzling aureole. The nimbus of glory to which heroes, kings, and prophets all owe their glory, superiority, and power.

"[Xvarənah is] of such a kind that will make a new world, freed from old age and death, from decomposition and corruption, eternally living, eternally growing, possessing power at will, when the dead will rise again, when immortality will come to the living, and when the world will renew itself as desired." Zamyād Yašt 19.11

Xvarənah (Middle Persian *Farr*) is the divine investiture of kings, guarded and released by Apąm Napāt. *Xvarənah* hides in the *Vourukaša* when an illegitimate ruler is on the throne, emerging only when a true king comes forth. In Achaemenid kingly ideology, the possession of the *Xvarənah* was the prerogative of kings from their family line. From Darius the Great onward, they all claimed to be *Arya čisa* ("beaming with the *Aryan Xvarənah*").

In *Zamyād Yašt* 19.5 Apąm Napāt takes *Xvarənah* to the bottom of the sea when Ātar and Aži Dahāka (the evil ruler/serpent king) fail to conclude their contest for it. This happens after Mithra, Thraētaona, and Kərəsāspa seize it upon the fall of the first king Yima.

In Persian epic, Mithra holds it in trust until Ferēdūn (Thraētaona) defeats the evil Zahhāk (Aži Dahāka) and reigns. Then Sām Narīmān (Kərəsāspa) gets the *Xvarənah*.

"[Mithra] the supernatural god who drives over all the continents bestowing Xvarənah, the supernatural god who drives over all the continents bestowing power." Mihr Yašt 10.16

Both Apąm Napāt and Mithra are guardians of the *Xvarənah* as the symbol of legitimate authority. In scripture, Mithra is a maker and undoer of kings. Apąm Napāt is the water aspect of this function, complementing Mithra's fire aspect. Kingly glory is the fire emerging from water. The taking of the *Xvarənah* from water by the legitimate ruler is like the taking of the sword from the Lady of the Lake in Arthurian myth: legitimate authority rests in the waters until the true owner of it comes to claim it.

The WarYogin must enthrone his higher Self in order for his *Xvarənah* to issue forth from the Cosmic Ocean within. He conducts a metaphysical search for the power of fire within his inner Chaos. The

WarYogin enters the water and returns with fire, with his *ātaršxvarəno* ("fire-glory"). Once the WarYogin has seized the *Xvarənah*, he is able to take on the Cosmic battle with renewed vigour and legitimacy.

"Behind him drives Ātar, all in a blaze, and the awful kingly Glory." Mihr Yašt 10.127

The *Xvarənah* is celestial fire and glory. It renders the WarYogin immortal and testifies to such through his victory. This is the luminous apex of his action.

The WarYogin's *Xvarənah* is what connects him to the World of Light. It is through his *Xvarənah* that he perceives himself to be of the same nature as Celestial Light. The Light of Glory endows the WarYogin with victorious and supernatural strength and consecrates him as a Being of Light clothed in sacred dignity.

His *Xvarənah* transfigures the Earth into a heavenly Earth: a glorious paradisiacal landscape. The incandescence of his victory fire sets the whole of creation ablaze. The dawn flames on the mountain peaks, transfiguring the Earth.

This is the transmutation of the material Earth into the visionary Sacred Earth. It is the psycho-cosmic terrain of the Inner Earth, the Paradise of Yima. It is the confluence of human and divine realms.

"May we be among those who are to bring about the Transfiguration of the Earth." Yasna 30.9

Yima and the Northern Homeland

"With his royal Farr he constructed a throne studded with gems, and had demons raise him aloft from the earth into the heavens: there he sat on his throne like the sun shining in the sky." Šahnāme

The primordial king Yima ("Twin") is the Avestan equivalent of Vedic Yama. His name is also cognate with Germanic Ymir and Roman Remus. He is son of Vīvahvant (Vedic Vivasat), a solar deity and the first sacrificer in early Iranian religion. Iranian Yima is not a divinity like his Vedic counterpart, but a culture hero.

Yima Xšaēta ruled over the Golden Age of the original polar homeland in the far North. It was a time with no ageing. No animals or men died under his rule. Plants did not wither, food and water were abundant, and there was no extreme hot or cold. As the population grew, Yima (with Ahura Mazdā's consent) expanded the earth on several occasions.

"And Yima made the earth grow larger by two-thirds than it was before, and there came flocks and herds and men, at their

will and wish, as many as he wished." Vīdēvdāt 2.19

The tokens of his royalty are a golden goad and whip – the tools of a cattleman. Yima is "rich in herds;" he is the first man, king, and pastoralist. His myth is that of a nomadic people.

Yima performs the first sacrifice of the primordial cow. This is the Indo-European cow that suckles the divine twins. Echoes of this mythos are found throughout the Vedic, Greek, Roman, and Germanic branches of the Indo-European diaspora.

The original Indo-European homeland, *Airyanəm Vaējah* ("Cradle of the Aryans"), is described as a cold country in the *Yašts*. It is a country in the far northern polar regions where "they consider a day to be a year" *(Vīdēvdāt 2.41)*, and "only once a year does one see the stars and the moon and the sun in their setting." *(Vīdēvdāt 2.40)*. This is the polar year in the land of the midnight sun, the extreme North where the sun never sets in the summer and never rises in the winter.

"I invoke the Glory of the Aryan regions." Vīdēvdāt 19.39

The *Vīdēvdāt* book of the *Avesta* gives a lengthy account of the land and the arrival of the Cosmic Winter brought about by Aṇgra Mainyu's creation of Aži Raoidita (the "Red Dragon"):

"The first of the good lands and countries which I, Ahura Mazdā, created, was the *Aryāna Vaējah*, by the *Vaṇguhi Daitya*. Thereupon came Aṇgra Mainyu, who is all death, and he counter-created the serpent in the river and winter, a work of the *daēvas*. There are ten months of winter and two of summer and even those are too cold for water, for earth, for plants. It is the middle and the heart of winter, and when the winter ends there are many floods" (*Vīdēvdāt* 1.2-3).

The chain of events that cause the cooling of *Airyanəm Vaējah* and subsequent exodus begins with Yima's fall from grace and loss of his *Xvarənah* for lying or boastful lack of humility. The first king and his land was brought down by an untruth or hubris. The fall of the land is connected to that of the king, just as it is in Arthurian grail mythos and Celtic "Wasteland" motif. The land and the king are one.

"And Ahura Mazdā spake unto Yima, saying: 'O fair Yima, son of Vivanghat! Upon the material world the evil winters are about to fall, that shall bring the fierce, deadly frost; upon the material world the evil winters are about to fall, that shall make snow-flakes fall thick, even an arədvī deep on the highest tops of mountains." Vīdēvdāt 2.22

As a sign of the king's impending downfall, Ahura Mazdā orders Yima to build an underground shelter, a *vara*, to protect humans from the coming *Malkosan* ("Evil Winters"). The *vara* is filled with waters and grassland. It is also connected to the Vedic *vala*, a cattle stall built to contain the Cosmic cattle: the cave that Indra and the *devas* destroy to release the cattle, the sun, the moon, and the waters. The *Malkosan* winters are like the three Germanic *fimbulvetr* ("awful, mighty winter") preceding *Ragnarök* (Twilight of the Gods). Following the downfall of Yima, the *Arya* migrate south in search of a new homeland.

The *vara* is built by Yima before he loses his *Xvarənah* and is described in the *Vīdēvdāt* thus: "And Yima made a *vara*, long as a riding-ground on every side of the square. There he brought the seeds of sheep and oxen, of men, of dogs, of birds, and of red blazing fires. He made a *vara*, long as a riding-ground on every side of the square, to be an abode for men; a *vara*, long as a riding-ground on every side of the square, for oxen and sheep." (*Vīdēvdāt* 2.33).

His Vedic counterpart Yama is the first man and king to find his way to the heroic paradise of the *pitṛ* ("fathers"). This *vara* is very much reminiscent of the Indo-European paradise of the elect, like Greek *Elysion* where everyone leads a "most beautiful life." Yima's "paradise" is like the Isles of the Blessed, which in Greek myth is ruled over by Kronos, Titan king of the Golden Age.

"The enclosure formed by Yim is constructed in Eranvej, below the earth. And every species and seed of all the creatures and creations of Ohrmazd, the lord, whatever is better and more select of man and beast of burden, of cattle and flying creatures is brought thither. And every forty years one child is born from one woman and one man who are of that place; their life, too, is three hundred years, and their pain and disturbance are little." Dādestān-ī Mēnōg-ī Khrad 62.15-19

Following Yima's fall, his *Xvarənah* breaks into three parts which is divided among Mithra (representing the priests), Kərəsāspa (representing warriors), and Thraētaona (representing cattlemen). All three are warriors, but this division represents the involution of Yima into the three castes.

Yima is called Jamšid in the later epic tradition. He is the founder of *Nowruz* "New Light" (New Year). Jamšid suffers the same fall through prideful untruth: he becomes proud of his achievements and forgets humility. The punishment for this crime of hubris is the dimming of his *Farr* (*Xvarənah*).

The *Zamyād Yašt* tells the story of Yima losing his *Xvarənah* due to his "consorting with the Lie." The *Xvarənah*, now in its deified form, flees Yima in the form of the falcon, passing from Mithra, to Thraētaona, to Kərəsāspa.

Xvarənah is pursued by Fire and the three-headed serpent Aži Dahāka on behalf of Spəṇta Mainyu and Aŋgra Mainyu respectively. *Xvarənah* flees to the *Vourukaša* where Apąm Napāt takes possession of it. The Turkic king Frangrasyan of Tūrān three-times dives into the sea to get the *Xvarənah* and fails as only an *Aryan* ruler can possess it.

"The Xvarənah went from Yima son of Vīvahvant in the form of a falcon. Mithra of wide pastures… took possession off the Xvarənah." Zamyād Yašt 19.35

The *Xvarənah* cannot pass to the Serpent King Aži Dahāka, who is associated with the Semitic language-speaking Near Eastern people in the *Dēnkard* section of the *Avesta*, as he is not a legitimate ruler. He chases the *Xvarənah*, but it remains out of his grasp. Aži Dahāka supplants Yima and rules for a thousand years before being defeated.

He is portrayed as the first in a long line of Semitic and Turkic enemies of the Iranians. The Dēnkard has Dahāg (Aži Dahāka) as the inventor of Judaism and the founder of Jerusalem. As Zahhāk he is ruler of Jerusalem in the *Šahnāme*. He is called an "Arab" in the *Garšaspname*. In the epics Aži Dahāka is imprisoned forever by Ferēdūn (Thraētaona), who wields the cow-headed mace or *gurz* (*vazra*).

In the earlier scripture, Aži Dahāka is more properly a serpent slain by Thraētaona with the *vaēdha* (javelin). The *Ābān Yašt* takes up the story where Thraētaona offers a sacrifice of a hundred male horses, a thousand oxen, and ten thousand lambs to Anāhitā so she grants him the boon of being able to overcome Aži Dahāka and take his wives. In doing so, he is asking the water maiden to give him the *Xvarənah* (a token of legitimate rulership), much like the sword from the Lady of the Lake in Arthurian myth.

"He begged of her a boon, saying: 'Grant me this, O good, most beneficent Arədvī Sūrā Anāhitā! that I may overcome Aži Dahāka, the three-mouthed, the three-headed, the six-eyed, who has a thousand senses, that most powerful, fiendish Druj, that demon, baleful to the world, the strongest Druj that Aŋra Mainyu created against the material world, to destroy the world of the good principle.'" Ābān Yašt 5.34

The king is the complete man, embodying the characteristics of the three castes: priest, warrior, and yeoman. Yima Xšaēta began consorting with the Lie, so his royal crown of glory broke up into its tripartite instalments. The complete ruler embodies the whole of the community. If he falters he loses the right to rule; thus, the WarYogin also embodies the traits of the three castes – and if he falters, loses his Self-rulership.

The priestly crimes bringing about the fall are impiety, unjustness, and sacrilege. Those of the warrior are cowardice, underhandedness, and un-warrior-like behaviour. Those of the yeoman are covetousness, venality, and adultery.

Yima, before his fall was the "mirror of God" – the microcosmic god. He was able to command the *daēvas* to lift his throne to the heavens. So too the WarYogin traverses the seven heavenly spheres to access Mithra's wheel at the pole and move the stars, taking fate into his own right hand. He keeps his sense of propriety, avoiding the crimes of the king and the high crime of hubris, thereby preventing his fall.

"The vile, through provision with temporary enjoyment — even that enjoyment of improprieties for which eventually there is hell — then enjoy themselves therein temporarily, and lustfully on account of selfishness; those various actions also, through which there would be a way to heaven, they do not trouble themselves with." Dādēstān ī Dēnīg 6.8

The Manifold Soul

"The body is material. Vital breath is tied to the wind and inhaling and exhaling of breath. The soul, together with perception, is on the body and hears, sees, speaks, and knows. The form resides in the sun station. The fravahr waits before Ohrmazd the Lord. He fashioned it because when men die during the onslaught of evil, their bodies join the earth, their vital breath joins the wind, and their forms join the sun, but their souls join the fravahr, so that the demons cannot destroy the souls." Bundahišn 3.15

The Cosmos and what lies beyond it have *gētīg* ("material") and *mēnōg* ("spiritual") elements. Form and formlessness coexist in a mixed state. This is not only the case for the planes of existence and non-existence, but also the life inhabiting these spaces. Both gods and men have *gētīg* and *mēnōg* components at the same time, meaning within the human form and detached from it are physical and non-physical parts.

The human being is composed of the *tān* ("body"), *gyān* ("vital breath"), *dānišn* (faculty of "knowledge"), *ēvēnag* ("form"), and the *ruwān* or *urvan* (eschatological "soul"). The *Dēnkard* states the body takes its form due to *čihr* ("nature" or "seed"), and powers of the soul find their unity in the *waxš* or *axw* ("essence"). *Čihr* and *Fravaši* (eternal spiritual tutelary) are agents of natural necessity. *Waxš* is a transcendental ruling force of the soul and motive power of growth and becoming: the agent of voluntary action.

"The ruwān is the master and sovereign over the body as the householder over the house and the rider over the horse. It is the organiser of the body." Dēnkard 3.218

The *Dēnkard* says that pure *waxš* is "the specific essence of man." *Ruwān, waxš*, and *čihr* are all *mēnōg*. *Ruwān* has *stī* (existence), whereas *waxš* resides within a thing that has existence. *Waxš* is the *nērōg* (force) within the *ruwān*.

During a man's life, *waxš* is mixed with bodily forces, but becomes pure again when liberated from the body by death. *Tān* (which means body) is connected intimately to *gyān*, the animating principle. Made of heat and Light, the *gyān* disappears with the death of the body.

Next in the chain is *ruwān* or *urvān*, the principle of immortality, which in another paradigm absorbs the role of *bōy* ("consciousness" or "perception"). *Bōy* is in the body, but not rooted in it as intimately as the *gyān*. It is not necessarily a part of the soul either, but a free force within the body.

"When the body goes to sleep, the vital soul is in the body, the ruwān is outside, and the consciousness acts as a messenger between them. It receives information from the ruwān,

transmits it to the vital soul, which then passes it on to the intelligence, the guardian." Wizīdagīhā ī Zādspram 30.32

According to the *Wizīdagīhā ī Zādspram*, the eschatological soul is subdivided into three parts. The *ruwān ī andartan* ("soul which is in the body") or *ruwān ī tanīg* ("corporal soul") is the *gētīg* form of the soul that abides with the body. The *ruwān ī bērōn* ("external soul") occupies the liminal space between form and formless states: it is the soul at work in dreams.

Wizīdagīhā ī Zādspram 29.8 states: "When the body is asleep, the *ruwān* goes out; whether this be far or near, it goes out and considers things. At the moment of awakening it returns to the body."

The *ruwān ī pad mēnōgān axwān* is the "soul which is in the world of the *mēnōg*" – this is the formless soul united with the *daēnā* and *Fravaši* for all eternity.

This last *ruwān* is the "soul," which is judged and passes over to the afterlife. This *ruwān* tarries near the body for three days before being conveyed to *Činvatō Pərətu* ("Requiter's Bridge" or "Bridge of the Separator") on *Harā Bərəzaitī* (Celestial Mountain) by the wind god Vayu.

Here, the *ruwān* is judged by Mithra, Sraoša, and Rašnu. After this trial by fire and molten metal, the *ruwān* meets the *daēnā* (female celestial double) on the *Činvatō Pərətu*. Her beauty or ugliness is determined by his earthly actions.

"And it seems to him as if his own conscience were advancing to him in that wind, in the shape of a maiden fair, bright, white-armed, strong, tall-formed, high-standing, thick-breasted, beautiful of body, noble, of a glorious seed, of the size of a maid in her fifteenth year, as fair as the fairest things in the world." Hādōxt Nask 2.9

If the thoughts, words, and deeds of the man attached to the *ruwān* have been good, if he has fought for the Light, then his *daēnā* or *dēn* comes to him in the form of a beautiful maiden and leads him to the *asar-rōšnīh* ("place of Light") or *Garōdəmāna* ("Abode of Hymns"). If his actions have been wicked and aided the powers of Darkness, his *daēnā* appears as an ugly crone. The bridge narrows to the width of the edge of a blade, and the *ruwān* falls in the grip of his hideous *daēna* into the demonic world of Ahriman.

The *daēnā* is a spiritual double involved in an individual's moral decisions. It is extrinsic to the body of man while he is alive during his earthly existence, operating on his behalf in the spiritual realm. *Daēnā* is the celestial transcendent "I" and divine feminine principle: Śakti, the "heavenly maiden" of the Indic tradition. *Daēnā* is squarely in the *mēnōg* realm, whereas the tripartite *ruwān* occupies both *gētīg* and *mēnōg* and the liminal space between the two.

"The body is mortal, but the soul does not pass away. Do good, for the soul really is, not the body; spirit really is, not matter. Out of respect for the body do not neglect your soul; and do not, out of respect for anyone, forget that the things of this

world are transitory. Desire nothing that will bring Penance on your body and punishment on your soul. Do not, out of affection for anyone, neglect the respect due to your soul so that you may not have to suffer a grievous punishment against your will." Sayings of Ādurbād ī Mahraspandān 76-78

The role of the *daēnā* as psychopomp, leader of the soul in the beyond, is described in detail in the *Hādōxt Nask* and *Vīdēvdāt*. It is at the same time situated both within man and outside him, when serving as his extra-terrestrial guide. *Daēnā* is related to the Vedic goddess of dawn, Uṣás, who is associated with Vedic Mitrá.

Daēnā – and her luminous nature – is an aspect of the Indo-Iranian Dawn Goddess. *Daēnā* is the *Somāteleion* ("Perfect Body") in the later Greco-Iranian Liturgy of Mithra. She is the "Perfect Nature" in Iranian Islamic Illuminationism.

The *daēnā* is not a guardian angel but rather the guide. She is literally "vision" – the one best qualified to see paths along which she guides the soul. The *daēnā* is placed on top, above lower forms of the soul as one of the *yazata* (gods) in the *Vīdēvdāt*. The *daēnā* is outside of man yet also part of him, much like his other purely *mēnōg* component: his *Fravaṣi*.

Fravaṣi

"At the spiritual top of the human being there are his three immortal 'souls': the daēnā/dēn, the frauuaṣi/frawahr (frawaš),

and the uruuan/ruwān." Philippe Gignoux, *Man and Cosmos in Ancient Iran*

The *Fravaši* is the genius or *daímon*; the male celestial principle of the *ruwān*. It is the Spirit: the divine spark within man. *Fravašis* are warrior spirits, particularly vigorous in warriors on earth. They are the transcendental personification of the fighting spirit.

As man has free will, so do the *Fravašis*. At the beginning of Creation, Ohrmazd offered the *Fravašis* a choice of whether or not they wanted to come to earth and do battle against Ahriman. They chose to come, setting the Cosmic War in motion, which in turn leads to the *Frašōkərəti* (Final Battle).

Fravašis are in one aspect a powerful band of 99,999 deities. They are also ancestor spirits: guardians of the *Arya*. They are invoked and propitiated for their assistance in battle. The word is feminine, but they are not female.

Fravaši means "he who has been chosen." The *Fravašis* are those who have been chosen and have themselves chosen to fight. Their name implies "preeminent valour" and "hero." This band of powerful deities forms a 99,999 strong army of warriors who watch over the *Vourukaša* Ocean, Ursa Major, and the body of Kəršaspa the Dragonslayer.

"And the star Haptoring, with 99,999 guardian spirits [farohars] of the righteous, is entrusted with the gate and

passage of hell, for the keeping back of those 99,999 demons and fiends, witches, and wizards, who are in opposition to the celestial sphere and constellations of the zodiac." Dādestān-ī Mēnōg-ī Khrad 49.15-16

The *Fravaṣis* chose to fly from their heavenly sanctuary to protect the Cosmos from the onslaught of the *daēvas*. In the *Avesta*, Mithra and the *Fravaṣis* have a similar the role to Indra and the *Maruts* in the *Vedas*. In the *Mihr Yašt* Mithra is accompanied by the "strong *Fravaṣis* of the Righteous."

The Spirits of the *Aṣavan* ("Righteous" Men) form the horde of Mithra. Aside from military prowess, they also possess glory and insight. They are "mighty, wholly victorious" warrior maintainers of *Aša* (Cosmic Order).

Both men and gods each have a *Fravaṣi*. Even Ahura Mazdā has a *Fravaṣi*. They were not created by him; they are co-eternal, predating the creation of the Cosmos.

Each personal *Fravaṣi* is the Spirit – the Greek *daímon* and Vedic *ātman*. The eternal Spirit of man chose to come and fight in the Cosmic War. In the *Fravardīn Yašt*, Ahura Mazdā tells Zarathuštra it is the *Fravaṣis* who assist him with their *rayi* (insight) and *Xvarənah* (Glory) in order to be victorious over *Druj*. Without them, Aŋgra Mainyu would be victorious. The *Fravaṣis* of the Righteous "fight in battles surrounded by light" (*Fravardīn Yašt* 13.45).

"Through their insight and glory, the sun goes on that path; through their insight and glory, the moon goes on that path; through their insight and glory, the stars go on that path."
Fravardīn Yašt 13.16

Each personal *Fravaši* is the guardian Spirit, the Passenger, the immortal deity within. It is not affected by the moral decisions and remains able to act in the affairs of men after the man's passing. It is separate from *ahu* (the life principle) and *baodhah* (consciousness). Along with the *ruwān* and *daēnā*, it is one of three metaphysical elements maintaining an independent existence within the microcosmic landscape of the body.

As Philippe Gignoux states in *Man and Cosmos in Ancient Iran*: "The *frauuaši* are the collective souls of the ancestors, comparable to the Indian *pitaraḥ*, and to the Roman *manes*, as well as an individuality, part of a pre-existing soul belonging to every man, which ensures his survival and immortality."

After death, the *ruwān* of each *Ašavan* ("Righteous Man") is united with his *daēnā*. This pair is then combined to join the *Fravaši*, making the separate parts whole once more, forming the Body of Light: the complete original Self.

This ipseity is only available to the *Ašavan*. He who betrays the pact made prior to existence in this world by his *Fravaši* encounters a hag in place of his *daēnā* at *Činvat*. He is cut off from both his *Fravaši* and *daēnā*. His true *daēnā* remains in the celestial, leaving the man only a shadow.

"We worship our own soul, we worship our own Fravaşi."
Yasna 71.18

The *Činvat Bridge* links the centre of the world to the Cosmic Mountain. The *daēnā* guides the *ruwān* (soul) to the *Garōdəmāna* ("Abode of Hymns"), the Region of Infinite Lights. The *Fravaşi* is the ruling principle or the army commander, much like the Stoic *Hegemonikon*. It returns to the heavenly realm after the passage of the *ruwān* into the *Garōdəmāna*. Henry Corbin in The Man of Light states: *"Daēnā-Fravaşi,* as the pre-existential fate of man, represents and is the holder of his *Xvarənah."*

The *Aşavan* is invested with a *Xvarənah* which is fully realised when he unites upon death with his *daēnā* and *Fravaşi*.

In Vedic terms, the *Fravaşi* is *ātman*, the immortal Spirit. *Ruwān* is Śiva (the male principle) and *daēna* is Śakti (the female principle). In the Islamic Iranian "Language of the Flowers," the body has *ćakra*-like seats of "angels," each of which is represented by a flower. Arranged in groups of eight, these flowers are a system of exchange between the celestial and the mundane. The emblem of the *daēnā* is the 100-petal rose – the crown *ćakra*.

"May strength, might, firmness, activity, victoriousness, come to all Fravaşis of the Righteous." Afrin of the Six Gahumbars 2

Ruwān is Mithra, the masculine fire. *Daēna* is Aši-Anāhitā, the feminine waters. These are united at death by the Righteous Man, but the WarYogin fights the greater inner Holy War to achieve this before death and liberate the *Fravaši* during his lifetime.

The reward for the good man is the heavenly realm. That of the wicked is the infernal. Both will be resurrected at the *Frašōkərəti* where the souls of each are given final judgement. The WarYogin joins in life his *ruwān*, *daēnā*, and *Fravaši*, transcending the world and liberating his Self to join the Army of Light as a fully *atidevic* Being, bypassing the judgement of the dead.

He forms the Body of Light occupying the centre and casting no shadow: the incorruptible Body of Luminous Fire. In this *tan ī pasēn* ("final body"), he releases himself from the bounds of time and space. He can act or not; he is no longer bound to the opposites, able to see beyond all dualities.

"When the wind blows forth among them bearing the scent of men, these heroes recognise in whom is the scent of victory."
Fravardīn Yašt 13.46

The Cosmic War

"The troops of Ohrmazd have been valiant in struggling and successful in will ever since the original creation." Škand Gumānīg Wizār 12.75

From the creation of the Cosmic trap designed to ensnare Ahriman, men have been fighting the outer, lesser holy war against the external Forces of Darkness that have so clearly made themselves known in this fallen age. While the *Gumēzišn* ("Mixture") has mingled Light and Darkness, the Ahrimanic forces have begun to coagulate into visible and imminent agents of chaos.

The agents of the Forces of Darkness have always been adept at making themselves appear the same as others. They are experts in disguise and subterfuge; but the mask is slipping and they are becoming more flagrant in their actions. They feel strong enough to no longer conceal their true nature.

Even if they fight amongst themselves from time to time and appear at odds with one another, they are always on the side of Darkness, degeneracy, death, and decay. They will ever be opposed to the forces of Light. When the Final Battle of this aeon commences, they will put aside their differences to combat Light and Life.

> *"If indeed the Sun were not to rise, then the daēvas would kill all things that are in the seven regions."* Khwaršed Niyayeš 13

Ohrmazd made the world with its Celestial Vault of the Sky as an irresistible trap for Ahriman. True to form, Ahriman attacked the world through a breach in the Cosmic Wall. The assault of Ahriman was the first battle of the Cosmic War. This is the war between the gods and anti-gods. The war is ongoing, but Light is losing ground. Only once the Darkness is on the brink of winning can Light snatch victory from the jaws of defeat.

The attack of Ahriman corrupted the world, beginning the *Gumēzišn* ("Mixture"). As with all wars, there are lulls and flash points. The *Gumēzišn* has gone through four ages during its involution.

The Golden Age gave way to a Silver Age when Yima sacrificed the cow and portioned it out, creating a schism. His fall followed and the Cosmic Winter began, which in turn gave way to a Bronze Age. We are now in the darkest part of the Dark Age: the Kali Yuga. Signified by utter disharmony, the Kali Yuga has allowed the titanic dark forces to enter through the fissures in the Cosmic Wall.

> *"They cried about, their minds wavered to and fro, Aŋgra Mainyu the deadly, the daēva of the daēvas; Indra the daēva, Sauru the daēva, Naunghaithya the daēva, Taurvi and Zairi;*

Aeshma of the murderous spear; Akatasha the daēva; Winter, made by the daēvas; the deceiving, unseen Death; Zaurva, baneful to the fathers; Buiti the daēva; Driwi the daēva; Daiwi the daēva; Kasvi the daēva; Paitisha the most daēva-like amongst the daēvas." Vīdēvdāt 19.43

The great Cosmic Barrier has been cracking over time as the world has become desacralised. The Forces of Darkness seep in more frequently and with less resistance every day.

As the protective walls crack during the Kali Yuga, man has even fewer defences against the Ahrimanic agents. The world has become ever more infiltrated and compromised. The forces of disintegration become stronger with each age in the cycle.

In this dark fallen age, desecrated, terrestrial forces have been unleashed. They dominate the world we live in, darkening it.

Now more than ever, the Army of Light must assemble. The final battalions must carry the torch within them and fight great battles on the field of manifestation. They must choose to align themselves on the Ohrmazdean forces of order against the materialist Ahrimanic forces of chaos.

"'We offered the pact to the heavens, to the earth and to the mountains; they refused to burden themselves and they trembled to receive it. Man took it upon himself and he is unjust and ignorant.' That is to say, he wronged his own soul abasing

it from so high a rank; and he is ignorant of his own capacity, since he is the place of the Divine pact, (or guarantor), and he does not know it..." 'Abd al-Karīm al-Jīlī, Universal Man

Cycles could not occur without man due to his centrality. All manifestations of a cycle correspond to his relation to the Cosmos. By virtue of his axiality, he is the essential player in the fight for the fate of the Cosmos.

The human realm is central; thus it is the realm of combat. Because he is the intermediary between the Upper Light and Lower Dark, the demonic forces target him specifically as they strive to usurp the powers of Light.

Dark forces seep in from the bottom wall of the Cosmos. They make their way upward, infiltrating the world from the South. Ultimately they seek to ascend the Holy Mountain. This is to assault the Northern Gate, door to the celestial realm.

The *Fravašis* of men chose to fight. Joining the Spirit of the Sky, they prevent Ahriman from escaping the world back to his abode of Darkness.

"The spirit of the sky arranged himself against the Evil Spirit like a warrior clad in metal armour... He set the fravahrs of the righteous warriors, with valiant horses and spears in hand, around the fortress... that fortress in which the righteous dwell is called Knowledge of the Righteous." Bundahišn 6A.2-3

Destruction and Creation go hand-in-hand. The forces of Darkness are performing their function. They are necessary to destroy this current world so a new one can be created. Only through the destruction of tradition can the powers of Darkness destroy the world.

Just as victory is within their grasp, the Army of Light, led by Mithra and the *Saošyant*, will repel them from the Northern Gate and devastate them. Only Ahriman and a few of his minions will manage to escape back into the Lower Darkness to plot in the murk while they lick their wounds. This will begin another cycle afresh.

The forces of Darkness and dissolution do not realise they are fatalistically bringing about the necessary collapse the WarYogin is preparing for. They are accelerating the eschaton, bringing the *Frašōkərəti* (Glorious Renewal) closer. They do not know that they are speeding up their own demise, and the victory of the forces of Light and life. Counter-destruction is what must be employed to meet the Ahrimanic powers; the WarYogin must also become destroyer, laying waste to the Dark world in order to make way for the creation of a new one.

"But the path leading to that end is spiritual warfare. And the meaning of spiritual warfare is putting everything to work so as to repel the enemies or kill them. The enemies in this case are nature, the lower soul, and the devil." Najm ad-Dīn al-Kobrā, The Blossoms of Beauty and the Perfumes of Majesty 2

Violence is inevitable in the fallen age. It must be channelled by the WarYogin in order to gain personal transcendence and to lay the foundations of the coming Golden Age on this earth. Only a militant outlook upon the decadence of the world – as well as a warlike Spirit that conquers the inner landscape of the WarYogin's being – will allow him to attain the *atidevic* state in which he reaches beyond the material world, yet remains rooted in it by choice.

The followers of the Lie have continued the rot that started with the Ahrimanic deception. They seek to chain man to the material world and stifle his striving on the higher spiritual path. This left-hand brotherhood is at war with the right hand of Mithra; most of the world is under the alluring control of Ahrimanic forces growing stronger day by day. These forces have used the façade of spirituality to bury man under the dead weight of matter to further their cause and bring the whole of mankind under their yoke of counter-tradition.

"Ahriman is the power that makes man dry, prosaic, philistine – that ossifies him and brings him to the superstition of materialism." Rudolph Steiner, The Ahrimanic Deception

The success of the *ahuras* or *daēvas* depends on mankind. Whichever side has more human actors will prevail. The WarYogin is agent of Light; he must fight and cannot sit on the sidelines, as to do so would only aid the forces of Darkness. The WarYogin must strive to restore perfection to the Cosmos, knowing chaos will always return through the cycle of Time.

He fights with a pure heart, as victory without honour is unacceptable. The WarYogin is is *ahūmbis* ("healer of the world"). He is *Saošyant* ("strengthener, enhancer, fosterer, promoter").

Mithra mediates between Ohrmazd and Ahriman. Without Mithra acting as mediator, Ohrmazd would not be able to secure victory over Ahriman in the Cosmic Battle. Mithra secures the supremacy of Light and Order over Darkness and Chaos.

Mithra is the archetype of a perfected WarYogin. He is the primordial ascended WarYogin. The WarYogin is a warrior of Mithra fighting for the Light.

"Between the Power of Light and the Counterpower of Darkness there is no common ground, no compromise of coexistence, but a merciless battle which our Earth, together with all visible Creation, is the field, until the consummation of the Aeon." Henry Corbin, Spiritual Body and Celestial Earth

The Greater Holy War

"I return now from the lesser to the Greater Holy War... the war against the lower part of our nature." Words of the Prophet Muḥammad, Tarikh Baghdad, al-Khaṭīb al-Baghdādī 13:493, 523

The outward holy war is the manifestation of the internal Greater Holy War against the lower self. The WarYogin's higher Self is his Ohrmazdean nature. It is pitted against his lower Ahrimanic nature and the demons that accompany it.

Man has the free will to choose between good and bad. The WarYogin battles his lesser, baser self, fighting against the negative forces formed within and without. The WarYogin has already internalised the sacrifice; he must now wage the inner Cosmic War against the forces of Darkness to ensure the fruits of the sacrifice are accepted by the forces of Light. He must battle the Dark world within that he may live in the Light. This is the Greater Holy War.

Mithra is the Cosmic WarYogin, much like Indra and the Buddha are in the Indic branch. He is the macrocosmic reflection of the WarYogin's divine inner spark of divinity. Mithra represents *ātman*, while Ohrmazd is *brahman*.

The WarYogin works within the *gēhān ī kōdak* (microcosm) to bring the Light into the *gēhān ī vuzurg* (macrocosm). In the *Avesta*, *haoma* induces *maga*. This is the state in which man succeeds in separating his *mēnōg* (intangible Self) from the corporeal part of his individual, granting him power and spiritual vision during his lifetime, and not only after death.

The WarYogin pours the inner *haoma* libation to Mithra. He induces *maga*, bringing about *abēzagīh* ("state of separation"). In doing so, he is severing his Spirit from the *gumēzagīh* ("state of mixing") of Ahriman.

"Just as Ohrmazd is on high and Ahriman is in the depths, and their powers struggle one against the other in the material world, so too there are two winds within the human body."
Bundahišn 28.12

Two paths lie before man: the heavenly path of the transmutation of individualisation, and the infernal one of the dissolution of the Self into the abyss. The WarYogin must attain transcendence; it is his purpose – "the crown of existence."

Because the WarYogin enacts the Cosmic War within himself, he attains the transcendence of exiting the Northern Gate of the Cosmos, allowing himself to realise his place at the centre of the wheel of time. He breaks out of the prison designed for the Ahrimanic forces and ascends to the Ohrmazdean heights in the unmanifested realm of pure Light.

The WarYogin works against Time. This is not the cyclical time of the eternal wheel, but the restrictive, corrosive force that is our enemy in this fallen age. Time in this sense is the repository of Darkness from which the corruptive forces are able to take effect in the world.

While working within the framework of Time, the WarYogin is detached from it, both above and outside it. He occupies the centre of the horizontal Wheel of Time, the place where the vertical axis mundi intersects. Rather than remaining above Time in the state of a liberated ascetic, the WarYogin works in the world while remaining unaffected by it. He is faithful to the principles of restoring order and balance to the world in body, but his Spirit is already free from it, abiding in its eternal state.

> *"Universal Man is the pole around which evolve the spheres of existence."* ʿAbd al-Karīm al-Jīlī, **Universal Man**

The WarYogin works against Time, but not against Nature. *Aša* ("Truth") is the natural order: it is harmony. To deny this is *Druj* ("Lie"). The supporters of the Lie are the men of the Dark Age – the men bound in Time who continue the demise of the world. Those above Time belong to the Golden Age of Truth. They are ascended beings outside the material plane, who do nothing within the world.

The WarYogin works against Time to bring about the end of the Dark Age and reinstate the harmony of Golden Age. He prepares the ground for the forces of Light led by the *Saošyant* in the *Frašōkərəti*, the Final Battle of our Age where the forces of Darkness will be destroyed, bringing the old cycle to a close. To borrow a Sanskrit term, the WarYogin seeks to become *Mukta Puruṣa*: a Great Soul, free from the laws of birth and rebirth, able to choose where in place and Time he chooses to be in order to fight for Eternal Truth.

"Your Self is a copy made in the image of God. Seek in your Self all that you desire to know." Mahmūd Šabestarī, Rose Garden of Secrets

Man is *theanthropos* in his natural, primordial condition: a "god-man." He carries the seeds of the Golden Age within him. In order to sprout the seeds within he must choose between action and contemplation. These offer two distinct paths to the same spiritual realisation; both allow man to overcome his conditioning and participate in supernatural reality.

The path of the WarYogin is one of action. In following this path, he internalises the sacrifice and fights the Greater Holy War within himself. The Path of Action is not opposed to the contemplative path as, upon its completion, it offers the same view from the top of the Cosmic Mountain. Mithra is the guiding light on the Path of Action, much as the Buddha is for the Path of Contemplation.

War is a path to supernatural accomplishment and attainment of immortality of the hero if the spiritual element is realised. Glorious material conquest represents a ritual evocation of the conquest of the intangible realm within. Warriors who are faithful to the God of Light can transfigure themselves and bring about overwhelming victories.

This is *jihad* ("Holy War" and "Path of God"). Islamic *jihad* is dependent on its inheritance from Iranian tradition. There, the Indo-European concept of the Greater Holy War was sublimated into the Islamic tradition.

> *"The 'greater' or 'holy war' is of an interior and intangible order – it is the war that is fought against the enemy, the 'barbarian', the 'infidel', whom everyone bears in himself. Appearing in the forms of craving, partiality, passion, weakness and cowardice, these enemies within the natural man must be vanquished, their resistance broken, chained and subjected by the spiritual man. Only at this point can one reach inner liberation; which will then allow participation in what is beyond both life and death." Julius Evola, Revolt Against the Modern World*

The lesser war of the Indo-European tradition is the material battle against an external enemy. To fight for a material cause alone is not enough – men need a higher purpose. The Greater Holy War is the ascesis accompanying the material war. It is the soul of the external war: the struggle against the barbarian or infidel within. The warrior who fights the Greater Holy War does not die but becomes part of the Army of Light in the Cosmic War, receiving his celestial fiefdom.

For the ancient Indo-European, war was a perpetual fight between metaphysical powers. It embodied the struggle between the Olympian, Uranic, luminous, solar, ascended powers of Light and

Order and the raw energy of telluric, titanic, barbaric, demonic forces of Darkness and Chaos. All existence was a continual, relentless endeavour to free oneself from the control of the anti-gods.

"The fight of Nature-within against Nature-without is thus seen to be, not misery... but a grand meaning that ennobles life." Oswald Spengler, Man and Technics

The greater *jihad* is both spiritual and internal. It is the fight against the enemies within. The fight of the superhuman element against that which is instinctual, passionate, and subject to natural forces. Inner liberation is dependent on the defeat of these foes.

The Holy War creates the inner *Imperium* and brings "Victorious Peace." Victory is the outward visible sign of inner rebirth. The victor triumphs against the enemies within.

The WarYogin dedicates the battle to a higher power. He fights against the internal enemy: the passion for life and the ego wishing to obtain the fruits of war – which desires material reward. Instead, he rallies to his holy cause and dedicates his victory to it. The materialistic, earthly principle gives way to the immaterial celestial; the WarYogin is transfigured from above at the moment of victory, making him appear fearful and wonderful – invested in *Xvarənah*. He is imbued with a divine Glory, a luminous numinous glow.

***"The human body is the measure of the material world."
Bundahišn 28.1***

Catastrophe occurs at the end of each age. The world must descend fully to the bottom of the Dark Age before *apokatastasis* returns man to his pristine condition. The WarYogin ascends regardless.

He does not wait for fate to determine his return to primordial perfection. He is his own *Saošyant*, his own saviour. The WarYogin climbs towards purity on the upward Northern trajectory, battling demonic forces that he faces within.

The WarYogin battles against his limited perception and tears down the barriers of delusion. Mithra is his guide of rising consciousness that overcomes fatalistic forces through free will. The WarYogin self-examines the unconscious and irrational Ahrimanic forces within. He channels Mithra to mediate the Ohrmazdean and Ahrimanic forces at war within his Self to ensure the victory of Order over Chaos.

"They are the best givers of help in the mighty battles, the Fravašis of the Righteous. These Fravašis of the Righteous are the most powerful, O Spitama, who are of the previous teachers, who are indeed of the unborn men, that is, the Saošyants who will accomplish the Renovation. Furthermore, the Fravašis of others, the living righteous men, are stronger, O Zarathuštra, than those of the dead righteous, O Spitama."
Fravardīn Yašt 13.17

The Cosmic War is happening, whether we chose to acknowledge it or not. While the forces of Light have mostly forgotten about the holy war for the destiny of manifest creation, the other side have not. The forces of Darkness work tirelessly to bring about the destruction of the Light and create a Dark world in their image.

In this fallen age, it seems almost as if the Dark has already won. But it is exactly these conditions which are required for the final victory of Light. Just as defeat seems inevitable, the *Saošyant* will arrive to lead the forces of Light into their final, inevitable battle.

The WarYogin cannot wait for this eventuality. He must prepare himself to fight in the Army of Light alongside the *Saošyant* and Mithra. He must wage his Greater Holy War and transcend the mundane world, becoming a god-man capable of battling the Ahrimanic enemies of Light.

Only by defeating his inner demons and ascending the Cosmic Mountain within, can he destroy the influence of Ahriman within himself. Only he can send the archfiend into flight, back through the walls of the cosmic barrier to his Dark world of the lower Chaos.

"The one path climbs to higher realms, to self-sacrifice, or to the fate of those who fall with weapon in hand; the other sinks into the abysses of slave pens and slaughterhouses, where primitive beings are wed in a murderous union with technology." Ernst Jünger, The Forest Passage

The WarYogin triumphs in the Greater Holy War by overcoming his inferior elements and remaining dispassionate about the vicissitudes of war. Combat purifies the WarYogin, setting him further on the path to a higher form of existence. He transfigures his action, making it absolute and pure. Without being killed, he experiences death and wins the Celestial Realm.

The WarYogin obtains an invincible force and remains standing as others around him fall. He overcomes chaos within himself and survives the dusk to rise with the dawn Light of Mithra. The WarYogin remains supreme master of himself, able to go beyond all limitations.

The destiny that the modern world has created for itself is overwhelming it. Throughout this, the WarYogin maintains his purified inner state. He belongs to his own inner landscape that no enemy is be able to occupy or destroy.

The WarYogin fights up to the Cosmic Mountaintop where it pierces the Celestial Vault, pushing the Ahrimanic forces back into the outer Chaos, purifying his inner world. He also fights to purge the material world of Ahriman and then exit it through the place in the celestial vault that Ahriman entered, leaving the purified world behind him.

"O you good ones, profound, far-seeing, curative, famed, winning in battle." Fravardīn Yašt 13.30

The Final Battle

"And they will make a new world, freed from old age and death, from decomposition and corruption, eternally living, eternally growing, possessing power at will, when the dead will rise again, when immortality will come to the living, and when the world will renew itself as desired." Zamyād Yašt 19.11

The *Frašōkərəti* ("Making Glorious" or "Making Brilliant") is the Final Battle of this aeon that will bring about Cosmic renewal. The Army of Light will meet the Powers of Ahriman and put an end to the *Gumēzišn* ("Mixture") and bring about the *Vizarišn* ("Seperation"). This is described by some as an *apocalypse*, meaning "revelation" in Greek; but a better term is *apokatastasis*, meaning "restoration." The *Frašōkərəti* will separate good from evil and, after this, the world will cleansed of its defilement returning it to the *Vizīrišn*.

According to the Zoroastrian sources, this apocatastatic return to order – called *Frašgird* in later texts – will be initiated when the *Saošyant* ("Strengthener" or "Enhancer"), a saviour figure, is born and leads the people in uprising against the forces of Darkness. The earth will be covered in fire and molten metal. The followers of Truth will ascend and the followers of the Lie will be burned.

The Gates of Hell will open. The souls of the damned will be redeemed and given final judgement. *Airyanəm Vaējah* will be the location of the Final Battle

"On the earth, in the likeness of springs of water, springs of fire will arise in many places. For Ohrmazd created with water and will bring about the end with fire." Vizīdagīhā ī Zādspram 34.49

Ristāxēz (resurrection of the dead) will bring all human souls back to the earth, where they will go through a purification in a river of molten metal. The righteous will assume their ultimate perfect physical form, the *tan ī pasēn* ("final body"), on the renovated earth. The gods Ātar and Airyaman will melt the mountains to create a river of molten metal, purifying all people and separating the good from evil.

All will be given an ordeal of molten metal for three days. It will destroy the wicked and sooth the righteous like a draught of *haoma*. The molten river will then pour into hell and destroy it.

Associated closely with the *Saošyant*, Airyaman will reconstitute Gayōmard (the primordial man). The hero Kərəsāspa – who has been nurtured by the *Fravašis* – will come back when the *Saošyant* appears to slay the Dark, Ahrimanic forces. This motley band will lead the Army of Light, along with Mithra, to fight the *daēvas* and transfigure the world into a pure abode. The righteous will abide in Light, while the wicked will flee to the Dark outside of the restored Cosmos.

Finite time will merge with infinite eternal time. The linear time that has been superficially imposed on the Dark Age will return to the cyclical time of the Golden Age.

"And he appointed for the middle third the creatures of the world... And that third is for the place of combat and the contest of the two different natures; and in the uppermost part of the same third is stationed by him the light of the brilliant sun and moon and glorious stars, and they are provided by him that they may watch the coming of the adversary." Dādestān ī Dēnīg 37.30-31

The material world and finite time were created as a trap for Ahriman. Men were created as watchmen and warriors who will battle against the Darkness. The outcome of the battle is not assured, as men have free will. Even if the Light prevails, Ahriman will not be destroyed, but will return to his primal darkness and gloom. This is the Final Battle of this cycle, not the final battle of all time, as time is cyclical. It is the battle that clears out the dross, beginning the next cycle anew.

The *Frašōkərəti* was subsumed into Iranian Ismaʿīlī Shīʿism, and the Assassins called it the *Qiyāmat*. It is reflected in the Germanic concept of the coming of the wolf and emptying of *Valhalla* ("hall of the slain") during *Ragnarök* ("the twilight of the gods"). The Indian-influenced Tibetan tradition has an equivalent battle at the end of time for the sacred city of *Jambala*, Northern Gate of Heaven.

"They will remain the guardians of the world until the Restoration." Bundahišn 18.4

The *Frašōkərəti* is the battle at the end of each Age of Darkness needed to restore the Light. While Light will banish the Darkness, it can never fully destroy it. Light casts a shadow which waits and grows stronger until it is once more time for another generation of WarYogins to go into battle. The *Frašōkərəti* must happen on a microcosmic scale, as well as on the macrocosmic level.

The *Frašōkərəti* within is the Final Battle of the Higher Self to defeat the lower self. It "makes glorious" the immortal WarYogin. It is the culmination of years of skirmishes fought on his subtle inner landscape over the fruits of the sacrifice. After defeating the Ahrimanic forces, the WarYogin finds himself at the base of the Holy Mountain. Having fought his foes and cleared them from the sacred city lying before the Northern Gate, he must ascend and go beyond the bounds of the material plane.

"All the bodily world shall become free from old age and death, from corruption and rot, forever and ever." Frahang ī Oīm 5

The Coming of Islam

In 637 CE, the Rashidun Caliphate under the second Caliph ʿUmar ibn al-Khaṭṭāb began to conquer Iran, sending the last Sassanid king Yazdegard III into flight. In 651, he was finally defeated, ending pre-Islamic rule in Iran. Following the assassination of ʿUmar in 644 and subsequent assassination of his successor ʿUthmān bin ʿAffān in 656, the 4th Caliph (the Prophet Muḥammad's son-in-law ʿAlī ibn Abī Ṭāleb) came to power.

Following the death of the Prophet in 632 CE, there was a succession crisis, with some backing Muḥammad's father-in-law, Abū Bakr ʿAbd Allāh ibn ʿAbī Quḥāfa, and some supporting ʿAlī ibn Abī Ṭāleb. Abu Bakr won, but was caliph for only two years, dying from fever in 634. The succession created a schism in the Muslim world between the Sunni branch, which believes in the succession of Abū Bakr, and the Shīʿa branch who consider Abū Bakr, ʿUmar, and ʿUthmān to all be illegitimate as the Prophet declared ʿAlī should be his successor. The Shīʿītes take their name from *Shīʿat ʿAlī*, meaning "Partisans of ʿAlī."

"If the enemy is a lion, be it obvious or hidden, one should talk to a lion with a sword." Šarif Muḥammad

Further compounding this divide was the assassination of ʿAlī in 661, which ended the Rashidun Caliphate, replacing it with the Umayyad Caliphate. ʿAlī's son Husayn was then killed in battle in 680 at Karbala by the ruling Umayyad Dynasty of Damascus. These two deaths served as a rallying point for marginalised Muslims. Following the death of Husayn, Shīʿism went underground. Shīʿites secretly continued to follow the *Imāms* (descendants of Muḥammad) while outwardly professing to be Sunni.

Iran, despite being conquered, had the largest influence on Islam within a century of the religion's conception. The Arabs did not have the scholarly systems in place that Iranians had. The Iranians very quickly came to dominate the philosophical and logistical development of Islam.

This was accelerated following the overthrow of the Umayyad Caliphate in 751. In 747, the Iranian general Abu Muslim began an open revolt against the foreign Umayyads. He defeated them in four years, installing the Abbasids.

"Who washes his hands of life says whatever he has in his heart." Saʿdī Shīrāzī, Golestān

The Iranians had more influence over the direction of Islam from this point and the Abbasids built a new capital, Baghdad, closer to Iran. They retained the Iranian solar calendar over the Arabic lunar and kept the Zoroastrian festivals of *Nowruz* and *Mehragān*. They took on the role of successors to the pre-Islamic Iranian Sasanian Dynasty, adopting their systems of governance.

Sharī'a (Islamic law) and the codification of the Ḥadīths (reports on the life of the Prophet) both occurred in the Iranian cultural sphere. Iranian scholars drove almost every aspect of Abbasid-era Islam. Literature and language were dominated by the Iranians, who formed the majority of Muslims, greater than the Arabs, who had become the minority. The Abbasids were Sunni however, and persecuted the Shī'a minority in Iran.

"Love death, that you may still live." Ibn Sīnā (Avicenna), Recital of the Bird

Shī'īs believe the divine and infallible status of the leader is only given to one man at a time. This is the *Imām*. All Shī'īs agree on the first six, but in 764 there was a split in the Shī'īte branch.

The sixth Shī'īte *Imām*, Ja'far al-Sadiq, had two sons. Ithna 'Ashari Shī'īs, or "Twelver" Shī'ītes, believe the seventh *Imām* was the younger son, Musa al-Kazim. They follow this line to the twelfth *Imām*, Muḥammad al-Mahdi, who went into *ghaybat* (occultation) in 873, and believe he will return as a messianic figure. This is the current state religion of Iran.

Ismā'īlī, or "Sevener" Shī'ītes believe the eldest son, Ismā'īl, was the seventh *Imām*. They believe that whoever the present *Imām* is, he is the unique possessor of esoteric knowledge and can perceive hidden meanings in outward signs. Ismā'īlīs are derisively called *batiniyya* ("esotericists") as their belief system combines Islam, Hellenic philosophy, and Iranian mysticism of light.

> *"Wisdom and knowledge serve to guide the wanderers; were there but one road, wisdom would be needless."* Jalāl al-Dīn Muḥammad Rūmī, Masnavi 6.5

The Sunni Saljūq (Seljuk) Turks seized power in Iran in 1038 CE. Sunnis and ʿAshari Shīʿīs adapted to Saljūq rule. Only the Ismāʿīlīs resisted.

The Sunnis and Twelvers conformed to the unified Islamic practices and laws of the Saljūqs. However, the Ismāʿīlīs – and particularly the Nizārī sect – did not.

In 1090, the militant Nizārī Ismāʿīlī Iranian Hasan-i Sabbāh captured the castle of Alamūt in the Alborz mountains. He and his followers then cut their connections with the Ismāʿīlī Fatimid Dynasty of Egypt and dispersed themselves throughout Saljūq territory in Iran. The "Old Man of the Mountain" and his "Assassins" waged guerrilla war on the Saljūqs for two hundred years. Hasan-i Sabbāh was, until his death in 1124, the first of eight lords ruling from Alamūt between 1090 and 1256.

In 1501, the Iranian Safavid family converted to Shīʿīsm and gathered an army of nomads. They overthrew the Turks and installed Esmaʿil Safavi as the first Safavid Shah of Iran. Iran converted wholesale to Twelver Shīʿīsm and the Safavids imported Lebanese Twelver scholars to help create the only Shīʿa state in the world – that which remains today.

"The most evil age is the one in which the carpet of striving has been rolled up, in which the movement of thought is interrupted, the door of revelations bolted, the path of visions blocked." Šehāb-al-dīn Yaḥyā Sohravardī, Book of the Wisdom of Illumination

Ismāʿīlī Shīʿīsm once again went underground, but heavily influenced the esoteric Ṣufīsm that flourished in free-thinking Iran. Early Iranian Gnosticism continued to exist in Islamic garb but drew on ancient symbolism. Iranian Islam encoded much of the Indo-European inheritance. Five daily prayers, heaven and hell, piety, the bridge of death, the angels Herut and Marut, millenarianism, messianism, and apocalypticism, as well as ritual purity, are all pre-Islamic Iranian ideas. Shīʿīs believe that the *Mahdī*, the god-sent ruler, will come and fill the world with justice, an inheritance of the Zoroastrian *Saošyant*. While Sunni Islam believes in spiritual authority being given to the best among the people, Shīʿa Islam believes in a succession ordained by god: a vertical transmission betraying an Indo-European sensibility.

As Indo-European people, the Iranians attached ideas of transcendence and esotericism to the Islam brought by the Arabs. Islam in Iran transformed to a non-Arabic form embracing Ṣufīsm and Ismāʿīlī mysticism. The institution of *Ṣufī* brotherhoods took place primarily in Iran; the *Ṣufī* notion of *ʿerfān* (gnosis) – sublime insight gained through personal discipline – was embraced by Iranian Muslims. This more mystic vision is the form of Islam transmitted east to India and China.

"Again you ask 'Who is the traveller on the road?' It is he who is acquainted with his own origin." Mahmūd Šhabestarī, Rose Garden of Secrets

No matter which foreign religion entered Iran, the Iranian soul shaped it to fit the people of the Land of the Noble. Islam is the last of a long line of religions to sweep through Iran, including Christianity and Buddhism, both of which were transformed by the Iranians to incorporate ideals and concepts from the depths of the Indo-Iranian mythos. Christianity became Nestorian Christianity. What would become Mahayana Buddhism was influenced by Zoroastrian thought after entering Iran.

The Iranians have always retained the kernel of their Indo-European ideals. Today this remains in the Islam that was shaped by them, made into their own religion.

"The journey asks of you a lion's heart. The road is long, the sea is deep – one flies first buffeted by joy then sights, if you desire this quest, give up your soul and make our Sovereign's court your only goal." Farīd ud-Dīn 'Aṭṭār, Conference of the Birds

Ṣufī Metaphysics

"If you want to be free, delay no longer your resolve to set forth on the voyage." Šehāb-al-dīn Yaḥyā Sohravardī, Story of the Western Exile

The entry of Islam into Iran in the 7th century almost immediately created a fusion of Islamic thought and Iranian esotericism. Prince of Martyrs Imām Husayn married Šarhbanou, daughter of Yazdegard III, last Sassanid sovereign of Iran. The integration of fire from Zoroastrianism as symbol of divine love was incorporated into esoteric Islamic thought. Ṣufīsm celebrates the princess Šarhbanou as the symbol of the synthesis between pre-Islamic and Islamic Iran.

Iranian Ṣufīsm recognises Zarathuštra as its oldest prophet. This comes from the *Hadīth* (the sayings of the Prophet Muḥammad) which states: "Never indulge in hostile or irreverent remarks against Zarathuštra, for in Iran, Zarathuštra was the prophet sent by the Lord of Love."

Esotericism cannot exist without an exoteric basis. *Sharī'a* ("great way") is the exoteric, religious shell of Islam; *Ḥaqīqa* is the inner, esoteric kernel. *Ṭarīqa* is the radius from the shell to the kernel: it is the path.

There are many *ṭarīq* that lead to the *Ḥaqīqa*. The most trodden one is that of Ṣufīsm, which aims at the overcoming of the *nafs* (lower self) through *maqāmāt* (spiritual development). Ṣufīs seek *fanā'* ("annihilation"), a nirvana-like state through destruction of the *nafs*, a veil that must be removed in order to see the true reality. This is done under the guidance of a *moršed* (master) or *Šayk* (spiritual guide) with a line of succession stretching back to the religion's inception.

"How wondrous and strange the human heart, which no one can see, save the pilgrims of the Spirit, who are the pure in heart." Šams al-Dīn Muḥammad Lāhījī, Jābalqā and Jabarṣā

Until the mid-19th century, Ṣufīsm was practiced by a majority of Muslims in the world. Sunni Wahhābism (Salafism) is the key opponent of Ṣufīsm; from the 18th century onward, the followers of Muḥammad ibn ʿAbd al-Wahhāb have sought to destroy all that is outside of its doctrine, especially Ṣufīsm. Ibn Abd al-Wahhāb formed a pact with Muḥammad bin Suʿūd Āl Muqrin in 1744, culminating in the foundation of Saudi Arabia in 1932. It is from the teachings of Muḥammad ibn ʿAbd al-Wahhāb that spring modern fundamentalist Salafi Jihadi groups such as Al Qaeda and Islamic State. It represents the polar opposite of Ṣufīsm on the spectrum of Islamic thought.

Originally Shīʿa also disapproved of the *Ṣufīs*. This is because the mystics revered saints more than the members of the house of ʿAlī. With the rise of Wahhābism and subsequent Sunni abandonment of Ṣufīsm however, Shīʿīs came to dominate the practice.

Ṣufīsm, also known as *taṣawwuf* in Arabic, was strongly influenced by Iranian Buddhism, notably the concept of *fanā'*; but in other ways too with the *jihad al-nafs* ("struggle against the self"), or Inner Holy War forming a part of the doctrine. This is where the *Ṣufī* seeks to eliminate the I and immerse himself in God until only God exists. This refinement of the Self is similar to the Indic doctrine of *ātman* and *brahman*, where the yogin aims to yoke his divine spark of *ātman* to the highest universal principle: the Absolute of *brahman*.

Ṣufīsm is active, encompassing all aspects of living, and is applied to every moment of daily life. This results in *ma'rifa* (inner wisdom). There cannot be Ṣufīsm dependent on knowledge without action.

"The spiritual state of baqā', to which Ṣufī contemplatives aspire (the word signifies pure 'subsistence' beyond all form), is the same as the state of mokṣa." Titus Burckhardt, Ṣufī Doctrine and Method

The *Ṣufī* seeks Truth, entering into altered states of being though either ecstatic *sukr* (spiritual "intoxication"), or *sahw* ("sobriety"). Ecstatic Ṣufīsm utilises the practice of *sama* ("listening"), which involves recitation of poetry or music and the whirling utilised by dervishes. Sober Ṣufīsm utilises the practice of *zekr* (Arabic: *dhikr* – "remembrance"), which can use a physical movement discipline, but normally involves mantra recitation.

Ṣufīsm believes in saint veneration. This makes it more compatible with Shī'a Islam, which advocates the veneration of *Imāms* and "friends of god" through adoration at their tombs. Sunni

Islam does not believe in the veneration of saints. The Shīʿī disciple can gain divine grace through the *Šayḵ* in his lifetime, and after his death by being physically close to his earthly remains. A similar practice is found in Indian with guru veneration.

"There is, moreover, a tradition dating back to the Sages of antiquity concerning the existence of a universe having extent but different from the sensory world – a universe with infinite wonders." ʿAbd al-Razzāq Lāhījī, Gawhar-e Morād

Iranian religiosity has always preferred inspired guidance and esotericism to imposed formal legalism. Iran was forcefully converted to Twelver Shīʿīsm by the Safavid Dynasty in the 16th century. Under the Safavids, Ṣufīsm was seen as a threat to authority. It changed its language, transforming Ṣufīsm into *ʿerfān* ("gnosis"); outwardly reconciling with official religion, but merely changing the language of esotericism. This *ʿerfān* of Iranian Islamic mysticism is in practice and philosophy distinct from the Ṣufīsm found in other parts of the Muslim world.

Avicenna and Taʾwil

"He who is taught a certain road leading out of this clime… will find an egress to what is beyond the celestial spheres." Ibn Sīnā (Avicenna), Recital of Ḥayy ibn Yaqẓān 10

The 10th century Iranian mystic philosopher Ibn Sīnā (known in the West as Avicenna) championed the concept of a spiritual return to the source. *Ta'wil* ("to cause to return") is the mystical return journey to the celestial realm through various "spheres" or "heavens" until one reaches the *'Arsh* ("Throne"). That is, the Throne of God.

This *ta'wil* is a return to the spiritual Home. The Spirit joins its celestial counterpart, much like the *ruwān* joins the *daēnā* and *Fravaši* in Zoroastrian thought. This is accomplished by the *Mi'rāj Nāma* ("Celestial Ascent") through the Heavenly spheres.

   1st sphere – Heaven of the Moon
   2nd sphere – Heaven of Mercury
   3rd sphere – Heaven of Venus
   4th sphere – Heaven of Mars
   5th sphere – Heaven of the Sun
   6th sphere – Heaven of Jupiter
   7th sphere – Heaven of Saturn
   8th sphere – Heaven of the Fixed Stars – *Kursī* – the firmament
   9th sphere – Paradise of the Hidden Imām – The Throne of God – *'Arsh* – the Empyrean

"Finally we reached the summit of the first mountain, whence we saw eight other summits, so high the eye could not reach them." Ibn Sīnā (Avicenna), Recital of the Bird

These spheres correspond to the inner landscape of the mystic, with each representing a stage of awakening. By journeying upward through the spheres, the spiritual traveller is able to attain higher states of consciousness.

As the 19th century Iranian holyman Šayḵ Muḥammad Karīm Khān Kirmānī states in his work *Spiritual Directives for the Use of the Faithful*: "His body contains one handful of the subtle matter of the first Heaven (that of the Moon), and his spirit was made from this handful of Heaven; one handful of the subtle matter of the second Heaven (that of Mercury) and his meditative power was made from this handful of Heaven; his imaginative power was made from a handful of the third Heaven (that of Venus); one handful of the fourth Heaven (that of the Sun) constituted his consubstantial matter; one handful of the fifth Heaven (that of Mars) constituted his representative faculty; a handful of the sixth Heaven (that of Jupiter) constituted his cognitive power; one handful of the seventh Heaven (that of Saturn) constituted his individual intellect; one handful of the eighth Heaven (that of the Fixed Stars) constituted his soul. And finally, his body contains a handful of the subtle matter of the Throne; from this is formed his essential and fundamental reality."

The first seven spheres, also known by the Old Iranian term *kešvar* ("clime"), correspond to the seven climes of the Indo-Iranian Cosmos. The eighth clime, or "lost continent," is considered the "interworld" between the lower spheres and the highest. Called the "World of *Hūrqalyā*" in Iranian metaphysics, it is said to contain other universes within: boundless states of consciousness.

This eighth sphere is the *barzakh* ("barrier"). It is the treacherous interworld between lower and higher ones. This is considered a dangerous state to cross, as the fall is profoundly deep for those who lose their way.

"This vertical orientation toward the Celestial Pole represented by Hūrqalyā is determined by the idea of a descent, followed by a reascent." Henry Corbin, Spiritual Body and Celestial Earth

The ninth heaven is known as the "Lotus of the Boundary." It is here the circular *al-Arsh al-Muhīt* (Divine Throne) surrounding all worlds is located. The Throne is supported by eight angels in the cardinal and ordinal directions. Upon the throne in the centre of the ninth sphere is *ar-Rūh* (the Spirit). Thus, the seeker finds his highest Self seated upon the celestial Throne within.

This is not the final sphere, as past it is the *atidevic* expanse "beyond the gods." After traversing the ninth sphere, the visionary emerges from Cosmic space. The WarYogin must exit from the ninth sphere to become *cakravartin*: the Lord of the Centre who turns the Wheel of Time.

"Rebirth is for those who never succeed in purifying themselves in the course of these returnings." Abū l-Khattāb Muhammad ibn Abī Zaynab

Wisdom of the Rising Light

"Divine light spreads to open the path of truth." Šehāb-al-dīn Yaḥyā Sohravardī, The Shape of Light

Avicenna and his concept of the return laid the foundations upon which Platonic Illuminationists built their Cosmic view. Ḥikmat-e Ešrāq ("Wisdom of the Rising Light") is an Iranian school of mystical philosophy merging Islam and Avicennan ideas with Neo-Platonism (particularly the Platonic Spheres), Hermeticism, and pre-Islamic Iranian wisdom. Ḥikmat-e Ešrāq (also known as Eshrāqiyyah – "Illuminationism") is the Philosophy of Illumination by the pure Light devoid of matter from the *Šarq* ("Orient") of the soul. It is the metaphysics of Light.

The founder of the Hekmat-e Eshrāq was Iranian philosopher Šehāb-al-dīn Yaḥyā Sohravardī. Given the honorific title Šayk al-Ešrāq ("Master of Illumination"), Sohravardī lived for just 37 years. He was executed in Aleppo, Syria in 1191 for cultivating *bāṭin* (esoteric) teachings.

In his short life, he produced a remarkable body of work. The foremost of these was his primary Illuminationist treatise *Ḥikmat al-Ešrāq* ("Wisdom of Illumination").

Sohravardī revived Hermetic gnosis in Iran. He was directly influenced by Plato, and acknowledges the ideas of the "Greeks of old" in his books. Sohravardī saw the ancestral wisdom on the Iranians reflected in the Greek corpus.

"If the commanding light shines by knowledge of realities and loves the Wellspring of light and life, if it is purified from the filth of barriers, then, it will be freed from its fortress when it beholds the world of pure light after the death of the body." Šehāb-al-dīn Yaḥyā Sohravardī, Book of the Wisdom of Illumination

Sohravardī taught that existence is a continuum culminating in the pure Light of God. The stages of being along the continuum are a mixture of Light and Dark. He held that Light operates at all levels and hierarchies of reality and that it produces both immaterial and substantial Lights. Included in these are angelic intellects, as well human and animal souls and bodies.

The neo-Zoroastrian Platonist Ešrāqī ("Illuminationist") philosophy of Sohravardī is clear that the "I" of every self-aware entity is pure, immaterial Light. The seeker must travel to the Cosmic North, ascending the Heavenly Pole through various stages of Light and Dark in the ʾalam al-mithāl (*"Mundus Imaginalis"*). This "world of the conscious" is a concrete spiritual universe, not a philosophical or conceptual world.

At the pinnacle of ʾalam al-mithāl the seeker can see the Cosmos in the Northern Light. He is able to see the sacred Cosmos where others see only the profane world. The journey up to this zenith starts in the Darkness as if at the bottom of a well. This Darkness traps Light and conceals it; it is of the demonic infernal realm.

After rising through the Light, the mystic encounters a second Darkness. This is the Black Light – the "Luminous Blackness," the "Night of Light." The Black Light is the superconscious that rises from the Dark of the unconscious. It is the "Midnight Sun" – the initiatic Light.

"The direction in which we must seek this 'eighth clime' is not on the horizontal but on the vertical. This suprasensory, mystical Orient, the place of Origin and of Return, object of the eternal Quest, is at the heavenly pole; it is the Pole, at the extreme north, so far off that it is the threshold of the dimension 'beyond.'" Henry Corbin, The Man of Light

The difference between the infernal Darkness and Black Light is the difference between Chaos and limitless possibility. They are similar in essence, but only the enlightened can thrive in the unlimited possibilities of the Upper Chaos. The divine and demonic are vague until the WarYogin can differentiate between Night and Day. The Black Light can only reveal itself once exoteric Daylight has been extinguished. An outburst of Green Light succeeds the Black Light illuminating the Pole's approach.

Passing from the Black Light to the Emerald Vision heralds the completion of the "resurrection body." This is liberation of the inner Man of Light from the material body of the outer man of flesh. The Man of Light is held captive by the Darkness from which he must free himself. To do this the Man of Light must find his Perfect Nature: his Guide of Light.

Perfect Nature is achieved at the centre where Darkness is illuminated by pure Inner Light. This Perfect Nature is the Guide of Light. It opens the door to a transcendent dimension, making it possible to cross the threshold.

"Seize hold of the cable of the ray of light and rise to the battlements of the Throne." Šehāb-al-dīn Yaḥyā Sohravardī, Book of Elucidations

The Light of daylight is that of the "city of oppressors." The seeker must free himself from his material exile, using the inner Light of Initiation (the Black Light) to find his way back up the Polar Mountain to the Emerald Peak and reunite with his Perfect Nature, at once his parent and his child. This conjoining the Guide of Light with the Man of Light is the Zoroastrian joining of the *Fravaši* with the *daēnā* (called the *shāhid* in Ṣufīsm).

This Guide of Light also has an equivalent in the *Sākṣī* ("Witness") of the *Śvetāśvatara* and *Kāṭhaka Upaniṣads* in the Vedic tradition. *Sākṣī* is related to the *ātman*, the divine spark. To Śiva as male counterpart to the female divine force of Śakti in the *sūkṣma-śarīra* ("subtle body").

It is pure awareness that observes but is not affected by the material unfoldings of the Cosmos. *Sākṣī* witnesses all thoughts, words, and deeds. Like the *Sākṣī*, the Guide of Light is above and beyond time and space.

The Ešrāqīyūn ("Illuminationists") call the microcosmic temple within the *haykal al-nūr* ("temple of light"). The *haykal al-nūr* of the human organism has seven *latīfa* (inner heavens) resting upon each other with their own colours, each a seat of a great prophet. These are the equivalents of the Indic *cakras* – the seven subtle organs or centres. They relate also to the seven *kešvar* ("climes" or "orbes") of earth and seven levels of the sky in Zoroastrianism. The eighth *kešvar* – the mystical Earth of *Hūrqalyā* with its Emerald Cities – is on the summit of the Cosmic Mountain *Harā Bərəzaitī*, called *Qāf* in the Islamic tradition.

"'Travelling the straight path' means straying neither to the east nor the west, it means climbing the peak, being drawn toward the centre; it is the ascent out of cartographical dimensions, the discovery of the inner world which secretes its own light, which is the world of light, it is an innerness of light as opposed to the spaciality of the outer world which, by contrast, will appear as darkness." Henry Corbin, The Man of Light

Visionary *Ṣufī* geography and ancient legends tell of a marvellous angelic race that populate the Emerald Cities, who are unaware of the earthly Adam or of Iblīs (Ahriman). Like the *vara* of Yima (where the elite shelter to repopulate the world after the Cosmic winter), these cities secrete their own Light, needing none externally. They are illuminated by their own Light: an Inner Light.

Above the planetary heavens, the eighth *kešvar* is threshold of the ninth sphere, the sphere of spheres. The mountain peak of the eighth *kešvar* is the emerald keystone in the celestial vault illuminated by Northern Light. It is the original pure inner Light coming from neither east nor west.

The ascent of the Polar Mountain begins in the darkness of night. This is not just the night of the Self, but also that of the Age of Mixture, of the Kali Yuga. The journey is marked with vicissitudes typifying the states and perils of undergoing an initiatic test.

The Midnight Sun bursts into flame at the summit's approach. This is the sun of Spirit, the suprasensory sun – brilliance of dawn rising in the Pole and place of the Spirit's origin. This *Aurora Consurgens* rising at the Emerald keystone of the heavenly dome is the Aurora Borealis in the sphere of the Spirit. The Midnight Sun is the inner light secreted by the abode of the Self, of the *vara* within; it is the Light of the Golden Age.

"When he who takes this road can see himself as being in the shadows, he will then have understood that he previously walked only in the night, and that he never looked upon the clarity of Day. This is the first step of the true pilgrim." Šehāb-al-dīn Yaḥyā Sohravardī, The Red Intellect

The WarYogin is a stranger in exile in this material world. He refuses the yoke of its oppressors, who cannot realise the purpose of his time here. The inward experience of the vertical dimension gives sense to the WarYogin's presence in the horizontal world. He stays oriented towards the Pole, distinguishing between Darkness and Black Light.

He also does not mistake the exoteric Light of Day – which obeys the demonic laws of constraint – for the Rising Light of the Midnight Sun. He seeks the Night Ineffable; the night of symbols. This can pacify the dogmatic madnesses of Day.

The Light of Day represents the material trappings of this world, while the Ahrimanic Night is the infernal Darkness of the Abyss. Rational dogmatic excitement and irrational lunacy cannot compensate for each other. Instead, the WarYogin must seek the totality of the Midnight Sun.

The WarYogin rises above and beyond exoteric Light and Darkness, absorbing neither, rejecting both. He attains the inner light of transcendence. This is the Black Light: the Midnight Sun.

"This is precisely the mountain which the exile must climb when he is summoned at last to return home, to return to himself. He has to reach the summit, the Emerald Rock... on the threshold of the pleroma of Light, the pilgrim meets his Perfect Nature." Henry Corbin, The Man of Light

Both the Eastern, Ohrmazdean Light of Day (sunrise) and Western, Ahrimanic Dark of Night (sunset) exist at once. The WarYogin transcends these; he does not become the sum total of the two, but abandons both. He knows Black Light is not a mixture of exoteric divine Light and demonic Darkness, but inner illumination – he is illuminated by the Light of the North.

Orienting his Self to the Celestial North, the WarYogin rises, leaving his shadow behind him and ascending far above the infernal realm. He casts off his shadow, leaving it with those who refuse to attempt the ascent. He climbs the mountain to the Emerald Rock at the summit, gaining *cognitio polaris* ("Polar knowledge"). His Spirit returns Home to the celestial source.

"I left the caves and caverns until I passed the chambers directing myself to the Source of Life. Here I perceived the Great Rock at the peak of a mountain resembling the Sublime Mountain." Šehāb-al-dīn Yaḥyā Sohravardī, **The Recital of the Occidental Exile**

The WarYogin joins his Man of Light (*Fravaṣi*) with his Guide of Light (*daēnā*) so he can transcend. He stays out of the paradisiacal abode of the dead and vertically ascends, allowing his Spirit to break free. The noetic Light from above – ray of the sacrosanct that illuminates and purifies – guides the WarYogin's Spirit to the Earth of Light from whence it came at the beginning of time – and where it resumes its original form.

"Outward colors arise from the light of sun and stars, and inward colors from the Light on high." Jalāl al-Dīn Muḥammad Rūmī, Masnavi 1.5

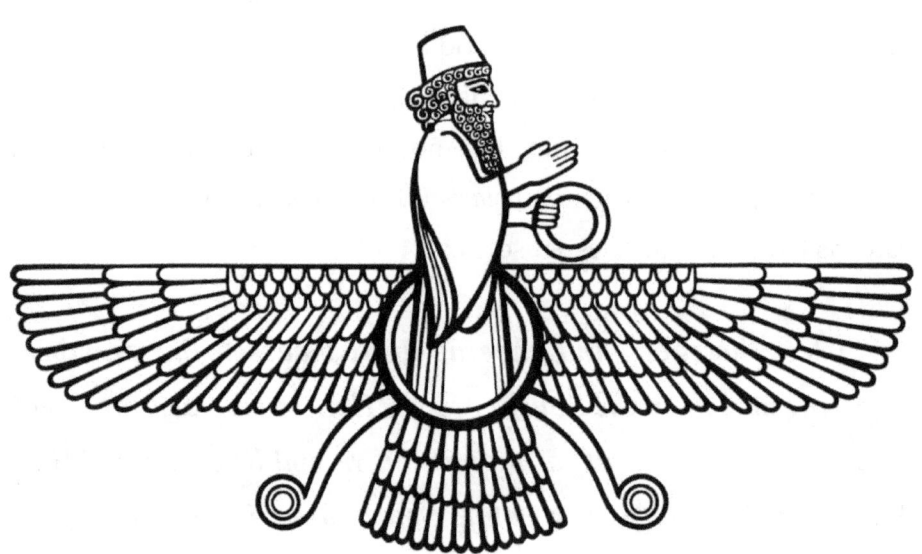

Luminous Night of the Emerald Vision

"Know that the soul, the devil, the angel are not realities outside of you; you are they. Likewise, Heaven, Earth, and the Throne are not outside you, nor paradise nor Hell, nor death nor life. They exist in you; when you have accomplished the mystical journey and have become pure, you will become conscious of that." Najm ad-Dīn al-Kobrā, The Blossoms of Beauty and the Perfumes of Majesty 67

The 12th century Iranian Ṣufī Najm ad-Dīn al-Kobrā continued the work of Sohravardī, elucidating the visionary experience of coloured photisms marking the stages of spiritual ascent. He taught that Light is in the North, Darkness in the South, and the Man of Light is captive in the Darkness. He must free himself through ascent to the Light. Kobrā says to first discern the shadow through spiritual warfare – to recognise the enemies and know them by name.

Stages of ascent are accompanied by coloured photisms: the pleroma of clouds the mystic perceives as he travels through spiritual states. First he experiences Darkness, then red (the seat of the devil), then white as infernal traits are annihilated. Blue is found as the lower soul surges upwards like water from a spring. The Man of Light is attracted to the green light shining from atop the peak. He must free himself of the Shadow, making possible the conjoining of the two currents of fire rising and falling to meet each other.

"Three adversaries disturb the innate knowledge of the divine; they form an obstacle between the heart and the divine Throne; they prevent the conjunction of the two rays of light." Najm ad-Dīn al-Kobrā, The Blossoms of Beauty and the Perfumes of Majesty 11

The three adversaries, according to Kobrā, are the shadow of Iblīs (Ahriman), the lower soul, and natural existence. Shadow represents the lower soul that must be destroyed. This is the personal Iblīs the mystic aims to separate from the Self.

After passing through the elements of water, earth, fire, and air, the seeker sees the colours green, red, yellow, and blue on the horizon. The other colours (which represent lower states) fade, leaving only green, colour of the Celestial Pole and the "heart." The heart is the homologue of the Throne or the Pole: the threshold of the beyond.

The Illuminationists talk of being at the bottom of a well. At the top, the Green Light is visible; it is attractive and terrifying. The mystic ascends to the light and at the end of his journey, seeing the well beneath him.

Originally dark, as the seeker ascends, the well is gradually illuminated, luminous with the Green Light. The Emerald Rock at the peak of the Cosmic Mountain spreads down, colouring it entirely.

"Green is the colour that outlasts the others. From this colour emanate flashing, sparkling rays." Najm ad-Dīn al-Kobrā, The Blossoms of Beauty and the Perfumes of Majesty 15

The journey takes in first sensory figures, then essences, then coloured photisms. Senses are turned to colours. New suprasensory preceptions can then interpret reality directly. Spiritual realities are displayed in colours, because the synchronism of colours and inner vision are now established.

On the lower plane the *nafs ammāra* (lower ego) is experienced as a black cloud turning to dark blue. This is the personal Iblīs. The middle plane is where the *nafs eawwāma* (intellect or "soul consciousness") is seen as a red sun. This is the scale which weighs upper and lower planes. On the upper plane is the *nafs motma'yanna* (the pacified soul), which is a green-emerald splendour punctuated with orbs of light.

The Man of Light frees himself from the crude ore of darkness, rising to the heavens of resplendent green where a star of reddish purple emerges. This is the intelligence of microcosm and macrocosm combined. Eminent scholar Henry Corbin says in *The Man of Light*: "The movement inward brings about the passage from this world to the world beyond, from the outer man to the Man of Light."

> *"Spirit does not cease to soar, to increase, and to grow until it has acquired a nobility higher than the nobility of heaven."*
> *Najm ad-Dīn al-Kobrā, The Blossoms of Beauty and the Perfumes of Majesty 59*

The *daēnā* (Guide), referred to as the Witness by Kobrā, is the heavenly counterpart who both witnesses the mystic's transformation and acts on his behalf in the heavenly realm. To the Ṣufī, the flame of *zekr* (meditative practice) burns away the Darkness and shadow of Iblīs making visible the *shaykh al-ghayb* (heavenly counterpart/Witness/Guide/*daēnā*).

Zekr destroys the *nafs ammāra* with fire. This is only possible with a Polar orientation. While the Ṣufī frees the Man of Light through *zekr*, the WarYogin achieves this through action – through movement. He acts in accordance to his calling as a warrior.

In Ismāʿīlī gnosis, man is an intermediary; he is a potential angel or demon. In the concepts of the 12th century mystic Muḥyī ad-Dīn Ibn ʿArabī, man is also intermediate, situated between Light and Darkness. He is responsible for both.

At the nadir, Ahrimanic Darkness is shadow: the negation or subconscious absence of Light. The Black Light is the pre-origin of all that is visible. It is the antithesis of shadow – the superconscious excess of brilliance, causing invisibility from being in close proximity to the highest Light.

"There are lights which ascend and lights which descend. The ascending lights are those of the heart; the descending lights are those of the Throne. Creatural being is the veil between the Throne and the heart. When this veil is rent and a door to the Throne opens in the heart, like springs towards like. Light rises toward light and light comes down upon light, 'and it is Light upon Light.'" Najm ad-Dīn al-Kobrā, The Blossoms of Beauty and the Perfumes of Majesty 62

Nūr-e siyāh (Black Light) heralds the threshold of the dimension of superconscious according to Illuminationists Najm ad-Dīn Rāzī and Muḥammad Lāhījī. It symbolises the most perilous initiatic step immediately preceding the Green Light of ultimate theophany. It is the Black Light of the hidden treasure that aspires to reveal itself.

Lower darkness is matter, while Black Light is absence of matter. The lower darkness is the realm of the infra-conscious, the subconscious. Upper darkness of the black sky is the divine Self in itself: the *nūr-e dhāt*.

The divine darkness of the black Heavens is the Black Light in which the ipseity (Selfhood) of the *Deus absconditus* ("Hidden God") is the Essence presented by the superconscious. It is spiritual super-individuality. There is an antithesis between the Black Light of the Pole and darkness of the material body. Subconscious Ahrimanic Darkness seeks to engulf the Light; divine, superconscious Black Light seeks to reveal it.

"He sees only his own Lord under the veil of the Spirit; then his heart is nothing but light, his subtle body is light, his material covering is light, his hearing, his sight, his hand, his exterior, his interior are nothing but light." Najm ad-Dīn Rāzī, The Path of God's Bondsmen: From Origin to Return

Bi-unity is not a union of Ohrmazdean Light and Ahrimanic Darkness, but of Ohrmazd and his own *Fravaşi*. As *Qoran* verse 24.35 states, "And it is Light upon Light." It is the joining of the Man of Light with his Guide, the *Fravaşi* with *daēnā*, the conscious with superconscious.

The WarYogin has to overcome both his own individual shadow and the collective shadow of mankind. The superconscious is spiritual super-individuality; it is not collective in any way. The WarYogin seeks not to reabsorb his *ātman* into *brahman*, but pass beyond to the *atidevic* superconscious state beyond.

Najm ad-Dīn Rāzī (a disciple of Kobrā) states pure lights and coloured lights refer to aspects of beauty. Black Light refers to attributes of majesty. Rāzī talks of spiritual individuality being triumphantly freed from the lower ego.

Then, the mystic enters the first of seven valleys (initiatory stages referred to as "spiritual states" by Rāzī and "centres" by ʿAlā al-Dawlah Semnānī). These are each coloured by a different light. The seventh is the valley of Black Light.

"What is corporeal becomes spirit and what is Spiritual assumes a body." Najm ad-Dīn Rāzī, The Path of God's Bondsmen: From Origin to Return

Rāzī and Kobrā map out the journey through the *nafs* ("soul"), *'aql* ("intellect"), *qalb* ("heart"), *rūh* ("Spirit"), *sirr* (superconscious), and *khafi* (transconscious) in terms of coloured photisms. The superconscious *sirr* and transconsious *khafi* (*arcanum*) are the final two stages of seeing.

Khafi is where the "time and space beyond" are revealed. The Black Light of *sirr* is the light of pure Essence in its ipseity, in its abscondity. It is the threshold of the Green Light of *khafi*.

In Kobrā's vision, the sun turns red in the black sky which leads to the Green Light. This Red Sun is Logos, Intelligence, Angel, and Guide. The Black Light of pure essence brings danger of dementia, moral and metaphysical nihilism, and collective imprisonment.

The Red Sun is the Guide of Light that leads the seeker on his journey. Crossing the Black Light is perilous in the extreme, but leads to the Green Light, to the *Visio Smaragdina* ("Emerald Vision"). This is the *šab-e rošan* ("Luminous Night"): the mystical aurora borealis symbolising True North.

"How shall I find words to describe such a subtle situation? Luminous night, dark midday!" Mahmūd Šabestarī, Golšan-e Rāz 125

Thirteenth century Illuminationist ʿAlā al-Dawlah Semnānī teaches of seven *latīfa* (subtle organs or centres) and their relation to *zamān anfosī* (psychic, vertical inner time) as opposed to *zamān āfāqī* (physical horizontal time). The mystic ascends upwards through vertical Polar time and these subtle centres – each marked by coloured photisms – to actualise the true Ego: the Man of Light.

The first is *latīfa qalabīya*, related to the subtle body marked with dark grey or black. Next is *latīfa nafsīya*, which corresponds to the soul and is blue. The third is *latīfa qalbīya*, corresponding to the heart, which is red. *Latīfa sirrīya* is fourth and corresponds to the superconscious *sirr* ("secret"), which is white.

Fifth is *latīfa rūhīya*, corresponding to the Spirit – the *rūh* that is centre of the "Throne" and marked with yellow light. The sixth is *latīfa khafīya*, the *arcanum* or *khafi* ("great secret") that is the *aswad nūrānī* ("Luminous Black"). Finally, the seventh and final subtle centre within is the *latīfa haqqīya*. This is the divine centre of one's Being: *Haqq* ("Truth"), marked by the Green Light of the Emerald Rock.

"Lo and behold, the Heaven of the sovereign condition and its power are revealed to you. Its atmosphere is a green light whose greenness is that of a vital light through which flow waves eternally in movement towards one another. This green colour is so intense that human spirits are not strong enough to bear it...

"And on the surface of this heaven are to be seen points more intensely red than fire, ruby or cornelian, which appear lined up in groups of five. On seeing them, the mystic experiences nostalgia and a burning desire; he aspires to reunite with them."
Najm ad-Dīn al-Kobrā, The Blossoms of Beauty and the Perfumes of Majesty 18

If the mystic stops at the Luminous Black they are in danger of believing they have become god. This is the delirium and insanity that can only end in reabsorption into the godhead. The Emerald is the doorway to *atideva*: the state beyond the gods.

The newborn higher Ego cannot look back or it will succumb to what it has overcome in a fit of nostalgia. It must continue on to the Green Light of Truth. There, the Man of Light is reunited with his Guide in hypostatic total reunion.

The theme running throughout all Iranian spirituality is light. It focusses on escape from the Ahrimanic Darkness to the Pole, which secretes its own Light. The WarYogin is a "particle of Light" imprisoned in Darkness. He must escape the matrix of colours to the realm of pure luminescence, where he claims his radiant *Xvarənah*: the Light of Glory.

"The 'clairvoyant' commits himself to the tarīqat or mystical journey, following the rules of spiritual warfare."
Henry Corbin, The Man of Light

The WarYogin scales the mountain of *Qāf* to the Emerald Rock at its summit, emerging above and beyond the natural realms. He gains the *čašm-i barzakhī* ("eye of the world beyond") so that he may see past the Green Light. He must pass beyond the *vara* of Yima, the Paradise of the North, the Earth of Light, the Castle of the Grail.

The Mystical Earth of *Hūrqalyā* begins at the Emerald Rock of Mount *Qāf*. This is the eighth clime, the interworld, and the *barzakh*. It is the barrier that must be crossed to reach the ninth sphere where the Hidden Imām lives.

The WarYogin must pass the form realm of the sixth sphere and the formless realm of the seventh. He must travel through the eighth sphere of pure time to the timeless ninth sphere, beyond all forms and colours. From the ninth sphere, the WarYogin can make the final leap to the *atidevic* tenth cosmic sphere. This is the Sphere of Spheres – the abode of the Cakravartin from which he may travel at will through time and space.

"Straightway lift yourself above time and space, quit the world and be yourself a world for yourself." Mahmūd Šabestarī, Rose Garden of Secrets

The Four Bodies

"It is in the astral body that the Spirit makes its appearance in the barzakh (intermediate world). This astral body is the vehicle and habitation of the Spirit until the 'first sounding' of the Trumpet." Šayk Aḥmad Aḥsā'ī, Kitāb Sharḥ al-Ziyāra

In *Ṣufī* metaphysics there are two types of body, which in turn are divided into two subdivisions. Šayk Aḥmad Aḥsā'ī, 18th century visionary and founder of the Šaykhī School of Twelver Shīʿīsm, best elucidated the four bodies. The *jasad* ("fleshy body") is the physical manifestation of the body and the *jism* ("body") is the non-physical. There are higher and lower forms of the *jasad* and the *jism*, commonly referred to as *jasad A, jasad B, jism A,* and *jism B*.

Jasad A is the elemental Material Body of flesh composed of sublunar elements. It is the crude physical body of the human being on earth that is prey to Time. It is compared to a garment worn and cast off. This body in itself participates in neither enjoyment nor suffering; it will waste away, but the person remains. As age wears the flesh away, the identity of the person contained within the crude vehicle of flesh remains recognisable. Similarly, if the *jasad A* grows through weight gain, the person remains unchanged within. It is the mere physical vehicle utilised in the material world.

> *"This world's body exists because of the soul which belongs to the invisible world."* Dēnkard 3.137

Jasad B is the incorruptible Spiritual Body formed of subtle elements. It is the higher form of *jasad* attained through transcendence. It is the *caro spiritualis* ("spiritual flesh"), or *caro mystica* ("mystical flesh"): the spiritual incarnation. When "the tomb" has consumed the *jasad A*, returning the elemental parts back to the elements (fiery to fire, airy to air, watery to water, earthy to earth), the *jasad B*, the "body of celestial flesh" remains.

It is the "clay" that survives "in the tomb," retaining its shape perfectly intact – the body which is "invisible" to "eyes of flesh." Like the gold dust in the crucible, it is only visible once the "waters" have purified it of the earth with which it was mixed. It is the bodily fire emerged cleaned from the water. *Jasad B* is "birthed in the tomb."

Jism A is the Astral Body composed of celestial matter. It is the vehicle that transports the Spirit through the intermediary eighth sphere of *barzakh* or *Hūrqalyā* to reach the ninth sphere and beyond. This astral subtle body remains with the Spirit when it is separated from *jasad B* at the moment of death.

Jism A takes the spirit to *Jannat al-dunyā* (earthly Paradise) or *Nār al-dunyā* (terrestrial Hell). There it awaits with the Spirit until the "first blast of the Trumpet." This denotes the "Cosmic pause" before the final resurrection.

At this point the Spirit and *jism A* are annihilated, constituting a similar purification as that experienced by *jasad A*. After four hundred years, the second blast of the Trumpet heralds the cosmic renewal. The Spirit is then resuscitated and reconstituted in the *jism B*.

"Know that Universal Man comprises in himself correspondences with all the realities of existence. He corresponds to the superior realities by his own subtle nature, and he corresponds to the inferior realities with his crude nature." 'Abd al-Karīm al-Jīlī, *Universal Man*

Jism B is the Essential Original Body – the Archetypal Body that is imperishable and inseparable from the Spirit. This is the fully purified astral body, which has shed its celestial matter. *Jism A* is the vehicle that allowed the Spirit to make its appearance in the intermediate world of the *barzakh*. Once it is no longer needed, it is purified and sloughed off like the flesh of the *jasad A*.

Jasad A and *jism A* are destroyed through the transcendent work of the mystic. They are the vehicles used to attain the higher states. Upon his death, *jasad B* and *jism B* return to the source where they combine to create the Supracelestial Body, the Resurrection Body, the "Body of Diamond" in the "aeon to come."

The WarYogin strives to pass beyond, leaving the Material Body on the Earth of Forms. Using the Astral Body to travel to the Sphere of Spheres, there he sits at the centre of the wheel. His Spiritual and Essential bodies combine into the Body of Diamond.

He does this in the present aeon, not waiting for the Final Resurrection of the Cosmos. He dies a ritual death, striving to free the higher from the lower forms before combining them into the fully-purified supracelestial Diamond Body. This is the body in which the WarYogin is able to operate in the coming Golden Age after the Final Battle separates the mixture, dividing Light from Darkness.

"Emerging from the last of these spheres, he enters the air in the pure state. His eyes gaze on everything around him; he breathes deeply; he is freed from the restrictions that stifled him; he gives himself up to relaxation in immense tranquillity; at last he breathes freely." Šayk Muḥammad Karīm Khān Kirmānī, Spiritual Directives for the Use of the Faithful

The WarYogin

"You wish to live, whilst I impatiently prepare myself to die." Farīd ud-Dīn ʿAṭṭār, Conference of the Birds

The WarYogin carries the weight of his ancestry on his shoulders, bearing the burden joyfully. This yoke connects him with the generations who have previously trodden the path he continues to walk.

He is unconcerned with the modern fashions and trends of the world. Being grounded in his ancestry, the WarYogin walks through the world, but is not part of it.

He operates within it, but does not succumb to it. He allows no temporal power to dictate the law to him, neither through propaganda nor force. He abides by the eternal Law, the Cosmic Order of Truth which does not waver. The WarYogin casts off the things of this earth, leaving them to lesser men who live only for material existence.

"Be single-minded among rulers and friends. Do not deliver yourself up as a slave to any man." Counsels of Ādurbād ī Mahraspandān 6-7

While the WarYogin has his roots in the past, he is not afflicted with nostalgia. He lives in the present. He ruthlessly burns away all dross that would mire him and bog him down in the past. He lives now but is not of now.

He stands upright among the ruins of modernity, rejecting weak mediocrity. He does not rely on ideas alone but acts in the here and now. He defends himself through the means of his time while maintaining access to time-transcending powers.

He is timeless, outside of the wheel of time and change. He remains steadfastly on his course. The WarYogin is the spirit of free and independent action. He is the elite who resists all automatism. His pure use of force awakens transcendent elemental freedom within him, rendering his upward trajectory unstoppable.

"He who follows the path of light Northward by the way of single-minded devotion to the Highest, passes beyond the manifest and the unmanifest, or subtle realm, and enters into absolute transcendence." Arthur Versluis, Song of the Cosmos

The world filled with the agents of oppression only serves to make the WarYogin's freedom all the more visible. It radiates out filling the aether that surrounds him with brilliant splendour – the aura of glorious victory. The WarYogin strives to transfer his *xwadīh* (Selfhood) into the *tan ī pasēn* ("final body"), his original luminous body of light that is incorruptible and eternal. He seeks to reside in the *abēzagīha* ("pure state") as a *stī ī rōšnīh* ("being of light").

The WarYogin remains true to his sacred cause. He is a holy warrior fighting a holy war in the hallowed terrain of his inner bodily landscape. His crusade is against his lower self.

The WarYogin is both Creator and Destroyer. Utilising *xwadāyīh* (sovereignty) and *frazānagīh* (wisdom), he combines thought and action, fusing them together into a potent force capable of violent transformation. He is relentless, ceaseless in his mission.

"For leadership over warriors there must be three (special qualities) distinct from the eight (of the priest): 1, a stalwart body with keen sight; 2, enormous strength; and 3, an intrepid heart." Dēnkard 3.223

He withstands the attacks on his Being, his Cosmic Homeland, from the deepest darkest depths of the abyss. These telluric forces are unable to penetrate the fortress of his Self. This he defends vigorously before taking the assault to the enemy.

Like Mithra he is master over death. The WarYogin died on the day he was born. He does not recoil in fear when faced with his death, but walks toward it with confidence, knowing his glorious end may come at any moment. He is ready.

Every thought, every action, every interaction is geared towards his transcendent undertaking. He wastes no time on impotent deeds that do not aid him on his path. The WarYogin's martial Way requires strength of body and mind. It requires purity of heart and Spirit.

The WarYogin manifests his violent potential externally, but remains tranquil internally. In the blur of action, he is steady. He trusts his Self, allowing it to take control during the flow state.

"The resistance of the forest rebel is absolute: he knows no neutrality, no pardon, no fortress confinement. He does not expect the enemy to listen to arguments, let alone act chivalrously. He knows that the death penalty will not be waived for him." Ernst Jünger, The Forest Passage

Active body, calm mind, and pure Spirit; at peace in a state of constant battle. The WarYogin is a blazing torch. He is a dazzling, blinding light that banishes Darkness, illuminating the world around him while conducting his silent revolution.

"Bow to no authority, but like the wind itself be wild and free." Šahnāme

Rostam

"From these two will be born a great hero, a mammoth-bodied man who will conquer the world with his sword, who will lift the king's throne beyond the clouds. He will extirpate the race of evil from the earth and cleanse the world with his heavy mace." Šahnāme

The greatest hero in the Iranian tradition is Rostam, son of Zāl, son of Sām. He is a peerless, invincible warrior. While he is first encountered in the epic tradition, his roots run deep. He is a reflection of the timeless warrior archetype of the Indo-European tradition, which is first manifested in the Iranian branch as the hero Kərəsāspa in the *Avesta*.

Kərəsāspa ("Lean Horse") is a pure warrior representing the warrior caste. Born of a dragon-slaying father, Thraētaona or Thrita, he is unlike his more reserved progenitor of the cattleman caste. A club wielder with cultic ties to the wind god Vayu, he can appear brutish and enjoys sexual liaisons with demonesses when not fighting against demons.

Manly-minded Kərəsāspa slew him. He took away the breath of his life-force." Zamyād Yašt 19.43-44

Like his father, Kərəsāspa is a slayer of dragons and monsters. He notably kills Aži Sruvara (the "Horned Dragon"), also known as Aži Zairita (the "Yellow Dragon").

Stopping on a hill to cook his lunch, Kərəsāspa finds the hill is actually the dragon's back. After running the length of the back for a day he brings his heavy mace down upon Aži Sruvara's head, slaying the dragon.

Kərəsāspa is most famed for killing the sea monster Gaṇdarəwa, who lived in the *Vourukaša* Ocean. The name Gaṇdarəwa is etymologically linked to the Vedic *gandharva* (celestial musicians) and Greek *kéntauros* (centaur). The "golden-heeled" Gaṇdarəwa rose out of the Cosmic Ocean to destroy all of creation.

Kərəsāspa leaped into the waters and fought the massive sea monster for nine days. He flayed Gaṇdarəwa and bound him with his own hide. The monster escaped, and captured Kərəsāspa's family. The hero fought the monster again, slaying him and rescuing his captives.

"Grant me this, O good, most beneficent Arədvī Sūrā Anāhitā! That I may overcome the golden-heeled Gaṇdarəwa, though all the shores of the sea Vourukaša are boiling over; and that I may run up to the stronghold of the fiend on the wide, round earth, whose ends lie afar." Ābān Yašt 5.38

Too proud and brutal, Kərəsāspa is eventually dethroned by the god Haoma. According to the *Sūdgar Nask*, an ancient commentary on the *Old Avesta* which survives in the *Denkard*, Kərəsāspa is tormented after death due to him smiting the sacred fire. It relates that when the dragon Aži Dahāka escapes his prison under Mount Damāvand at the *Frašōkərəti*, Kərəsāspa will be "roused to smite him, and to tame that powerful fiend for the world and creatures."

Garšāsp

"The brave hero rushed on with his heavy club, he came forward roaring like a lion. He struck him with such force and power that the blow knocked stones from the mountain. He took off his head and his brains mixed with earth and blood. This animal, mountain of combat, fell overthrown."
Garšāspnāme

In Iranian epic, Kərəsāspa became Garšāsp. He is first mentioned in the *Šahnāme* ("Book of Kings") of Abu'l-Qāsem Ferdowsī, the 10th century national epic of Iran. In this book, he is mentioned only as being a king of Iran and ancestor of the great hero Rostam. The mace of Garšāsp is passed on to Rostam in the epic, signifying the connection between the two heroes and indicating they are one and the same archetype.

The full story of Garšāsp, based on the Avestan mythos, is found in the 11th century *Garšāspnāme* ("Book of Garšāsp") by Abū Manṣūr ʿAlī b Aḥmad Asadī Ṭūsī. In this work, Garšāsp is the son of Etreṭ

(Thrita), king of Zābolestān, and a descendent of Jamšid (Yima). He is born when Zahhāk (Aži Dahāka), the serpent king, is still on the imperial throne.

Zahhāk meets the young Garšāsp while travelling through Zābolestān. The king tells him he should slay a dragon that came out from the sea and settled on Mount Šekāvand. Garšāsp slays the dragon, then travels to India to fight against rebels who do not acknowledge Zahhāk.

After putting down the insurrection, Garšāsp returns to Zābol and reinstates his father on the throne of Zābolestān, who was defeated by the neighbouring king of Kābul. He then founds the city of Sistān, fights in various battles, and becomes the king upon the death of his father. Having no powerful son of his own, he adopts his nephew Narīmān, the great-grandfather of Rostam. Garšāsp then fights another battle and slays another dragon before passing away, leaving the throne of Zābolestān to Narīmān.

Rostam

"Rostam rallied against fate." Šahnāme

No other hero occupies the Iranian conscious as Rostam does. He is the archetype of the holy warrior. Fierce, unassailable, noble, fearless, strong. He has become the standard to which Iranian men aspire. He is, alongside ʿAlī ibn Abī Ṭāleb, hero of the *zurxāne* ("house of strength").

In the Muslim wrestling *akharas* in India he takes the place of the Hindu god Hanumān as the spiritual patron.

While Rostam is not explicitly an incarnation of Kərəsāspa he is implicitly, being the consummate mace-wielding, dragon-slaying *männerbund* hero. He is, however, a more refined version of the archetype, unlike the more raw and brutal Garšāsp. This is particularly apparent in the tales of his deeds in the 10th century epic *Šahnāme*. The poem celebrates Iran's pre-Islamic past, transferring the Avestan and Vedic material into a pseudo-historical setting.

It is in the *Šahnāme* that Yima becomes Jamšid, Kərəsāspa becomes Garšāsp, and so forth. Deities are reconciled as heroes for the Islamic audience. The ancient figures are not made into Muslims in the work, as the book ends with the Islamisation of Iran.

"I am Rostam, the son of Zāl, who was the son of Sām, of the family of Narīmān." Šahnāme

Rostam ("Strong as a River") is born to the royal family of Zābolestān, an area now occupying southern Afghanistan. His home city of Sistān, founded by Garšāsp, was known in ancient times as Sakastān ("Land of the Saka"). This makes it likely that Rostam and his forebears were seen as being Saka (Scythian) people.

Rostam, like his father Zāl and grandfather Sām, do not lay any claim to the crown of Iran. Instead they loyally fight for the imperial Kayanid dynasty as generals and heroes.

A Herakles-type figure, Rostam is born to Zāl and Rudaba, a princess of Kābol. Due to his immense size this happens via a *Rostamzad* ("Rostam escape"): Caesarean section. Rostam quickly grows and is trained by his father in the arts of war. After slaying a mad elephant and sacking a fortress, Rostam becomes a regular fixture at the Iranian court and reliable warrior for Kay Kāvus (Avestan Kavi Usan), king of Iran.

He always rides into battle on his mighty stallion Rak͟s while wearing the *Babr-e Bayān*. This is a fireproof, waterproof, weaponproof coat that Rostam made from a slain dragon, tiger, or leopard. Sometimes called the *Palangina*, it is usually depicted as a leopard (*palang*) or tiger skin.

"The world was as I willed it to be, ordered by my sword and mace" *Šahnāme*

The most famous exploits of Rostam are the *Haftkhān-e-Rostam* (Seven Trials of Rostam). King Kay Kāvus, in a bout of pride, attempts to conquer Māzandarān, land of the *dīvs* (*daēvas*). The demons capture him and take him and his army as prisoners.

Kay Kāvus manages to send a messenger to Zāl informing him of what has happened. Zāl then tells Rostam to go to Māzandarān and save the king. This journey presents seven trials for Rostam.

The Indo-European origin of this mythos is deep. It ties to both the Labours of Herakles and the Arthurian Grail mythos.

Rostam rides out from Sistān on Rakš and after a day of travel, he lies down to rest. While he is sleeping, a lion spots him and decides to take down Rakš. The stallion attacks the lion after it charges him, killing it with his teeth and hooves. Rostam wakes up and finds the dead lion which Rakš has killed. This is his first trial.

His second trial is finding a spring of water. The hero crosses a desert with no water. He spots a sheep which he then follows to the spring where he quenches his thirst.

"No dragon, dīv, or lion can evade my fury and my sword's avenging blade." Šahnāme

Next, a dragon appears as Rostam is sleeping. Rakš wakes Rostam, but the dragon goes into hiding. This happens a second time, making Rostam angry with his steed for waking him unnecessarily.

The third time the dragon appears, Rakš wakes Rostam and a flash of light appears in the heavens. The dragon is revealed to Rostam, who then slays it in battle with his sword. As a result the desert is flooded with blood and poison.

As Rostam continues through the desert, he stumbles on a feast and lute set out for sorcerers who have fled on his approach. Rostam sings a song about his exploits as he drinks some wine, which alerts a witch to his presence. The witch appears as a young maiden, but Rostam is not fooled, handing her the goblet of wine and invoking the name of God.

This makes the witch turn black. Rostam ties her up and makes her reveal her true form. He then cuts her in two, completing his fourth trial.

"You should realise that the *dīv* represents evil people, those who are ungrateful to God." Šahnāme

Next, Rostam enters the lands of a young *dīv* lord called Olad. The *dīv* and his men ride out to see who is riding through his wheat fields. Rostam chops off the heads of the warriors and captures Olad with his lariat.

Rostam then tells Olad that if he helps him find his way through Māzandarān to the cave where Kay Kāvus is held captive, he will kill the Dīv-e Sepid ("White Demon"). Afterward he will put Olad on the throne of Māzandarān. Olad agrees, leading Rostam to the border of Māzandarān, which has fires burning on all sides.

Rostam ties Olad to a tree and goes in search of the Aržang Dīv ("Worthy Demon"), one of the chiefs of Māzandarān and a general of the White Demon, high chieftain of the demons. He finds the camp of Aržang where a *dīv* army are roused by the snorting of Rakš. The *dīvs* fly into a panic which wakes Aržang who rushes out of his tent.

Rostam descends upon him, ripping the demon's head off with his bare hands. He then slaughters the other *dīvs* before returning to untie Olad. The young demon then leads Rostam to the city where Kay Kāvus and the soldiers are being held.

Rostam frees the king. In doing so, he discovers the king and his men have gone blind from the darkness of Māzandarān. Rostam sets out to the cave of the White Demon, whose blood will cure the king's blindness.

"With your mace and the might of your royal farr you destroyed the demons of Māzandarān." Šahnāme

Rostam rides with Olad to the mountains, finding the entrance to the cave. Within is a massive army of *dīvs*. Olad advises Rostam to wait until the sun rises and the demons go to sleep before attacking.

When the sun is high in the sky, Rostam draws his sword, enters the cave on foot, and bellows out his name. Then he fights the demons. After an epic battle with the enormous White Demon, Rostam cuts out his heart and liver, flooding the cave with blood.

Rostam promises to install Olad as ruler of Māzandarān. He then returns to Kay Kāvus and brushes his eyes with the blood of the White Demon, restoring the king's sight. After an exchange of letters between Kay Kāvus and the king of Māzandarān, a great battle is waged between the Iranians and the demons of Māzandarān.

Rostam runs the king of Māzandarān through with his lance. Then Olad is installed as ruler of the land of the *dīvs*. Rostam is given the title *Jahān Pahlavān* ("Champion of All the World") by Kay Kāvus.

"Enemies are many and the years are few" Šahnāme

Rostam faces more battles and tests throughout his extremely long life. Some of these involve his formidable strength, but others require guile. Rostam rescues the Iranian prince Bizhan from the enemy Turkic state of Tūrān by disguising himself as a merchant in order to enter the Tūrānian territory and return the prince to Iran.

The most famous of his other exploits is Rostam's battle against the Akvān Dīv. The name Akvān is likely a corruption of the Avestan demon Akōman ("Evil Mind").

A herder comes to Kay Khosrow, the king of Iran after Kay Kāvus, complaining of a huge wild ass killing his horses. Kay Khosrow, who is wise and insightful, understands that the creature is likely an agent of Ahriman in disguise. He sends Rostam to investigate.

After three days, Rostam finds the ass. He then chases it for three further days, unable to catch it or shoot it. This leads him to recognise it must be the famous Akvān Dīv in disguise.

"Rostam twisted in the saddle and raised his mace, then brought it down with a blow like a blacksmith at his forge. The blow landed on the div's head and his skull and brains were smashed by its force." Šahnāme

Exhausted, Rostam lies down to sleep. The Akvān Dīv transforms into a wind. He digs out the ground beneath Rostam before transforming back into his demonic form and hurling the hero into the ocean.

Rostam swims back to the land and finds that Rakš has been taken by Afrasyab, the Turkic king of Tūrān. He rescues his horse, driving off the herds of Afrasyab, as well as killing many of Afrasyab's soldiers. Rostam then finds the Akvān Dīv and smashes his skull with his mace, the mace of Garšāsp.

Rostam is the Scythian wolf warrior doing battle as Mithra's agent with his invulnerable dragon skin armour, and smashing *daēvas'* skulls with his ox-headed mace. His banner carried the dragon device, much as the Scythians carried the wolf totem into battle. Dragon and wolf are intrinsically intertwined in mythic imagery. He is a more refined *männerbund* hero: a noble wolf.

This invulnerable hero is eventually brought down by his own half-brother by deception. Unable to defeat him in open combat, Shaghad, son of Zāl, conspires to trick Rostam into falling into a pit filled with poisoned spears. As his last act, Rostam fires an arrow at Shaghad, killing him before expiring and avenging his own death.

"If I live today, I shall live forever." Šahnāme

Ḥosayn-e Kord

The medieval period of Iran brought one further reflection of the Rostam heritage. The tale of Ḥosayn-e Kord-e Šabestari is of a Kurdish warrior from Šabestar in East Azerbaijan Province in Iran. He displays many Rostam-like traits.

The only surviving manuscript of the Persian romance of Ḥosayn-e Kord is from the 19th century, but set in the 16th century. Like that of Rostam, the content of the tale harkens back to deep Indo-Iranian antiquity. The identification with him as a Kord ("Kurd") is likely a corruption of the Classical Persian word *gord*, meaning "courageous" or "brave."

The story starts when the governor of Tabriz attacks the city of Balḵ in Afghanistan. The governor of Balḵ turns to the Mongolian emperor of Ḵeṭā for assistance. The Mongolian emperor sends two warriors and their soldiers to Tabriz and Eṣfahān in Iran with the aim of deposing the Safavid Šāh ʿAbbās.

Babrāz Khan, one of the Mongolians, begins to terrorise the city of Tabriz when the hero Ḥosayn suddenly appears and defeats the Mongols and saves Šāh ʿAbbās. He then travels to India, embarking on various adventures and challenges including fighting a sea monster like Kərəsāspa. He battles giants, dragons, ghosts, and witches, travelling to a frozen island in the far North before returning to Iran.

"Ḥosein matures in terms of martial training, yet in terms of social sensitivity he stays unrefined throughout his life. His sole true concern is his own independence, and only when forced by inevitable necessity does he acknowledge the superiority of his masters." Ulrich Marzolph, The Persian Popular Romance Ḥosein-e Kord

Ḥosayn displays several Indo-European wolf warrior characteristics. He wields a club and goes into the berserk state several times, biting himself before entering into a rage that makes the world dark. Ḥosayn is strong, fearless, and valiant from the very beginning. He embodies the Indo-European hero who devotes his life to fighting for justice.

Ḥosayn is explicitly linked in the story with the *'ayyāran* ("helpers"). These were sworn brothers descended from aristocratic Sassanian "horsemen," or knights errant who typified *javānmardi* ("nobility" or "chivalry"). Ḥosayn exemplifies the *'ayyāran*, who in other stories are associated with virility, mania, and wolves.

"The lion has returned from victory; dark is the heart now of his enemy." Šahnāme

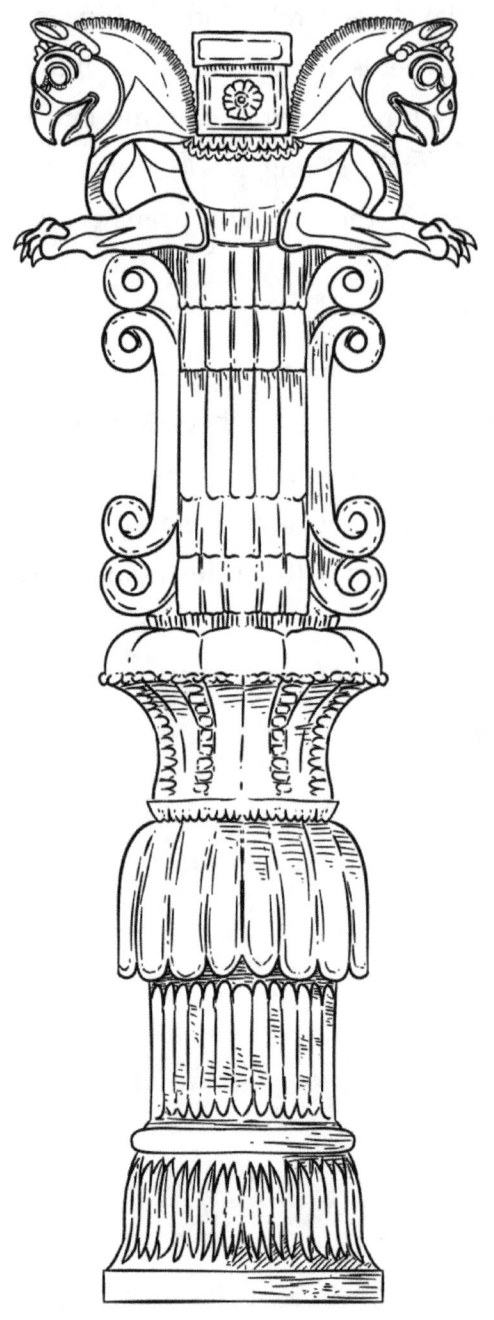

Part II: Practice

Pahlavāni and Javānmardi

"O young man... do not become without fervour in counter-attack owing to your blissful happiness" Inscription of Darius I at Naqš-e Rostam

Two intrinsically interlinked concepts form the basis of the Iranian warrior ethos. *Pahlavāni* ("heroism") and *javānmardi* ("nobility") are used almost interchangeably to denote the chivalric concept at the heart of the noble warrior band. *Pahlavāni* is also a name given to the sport practiced in the *zurxāne* ("house of strength"), where both terms are used to denote the character of the man who trains in the ancient sport.

Pahlavān (plural *pahlavānān*) in its most simple definition means "hero," and denotes a strong, athletic man: a paladin, champion, army commander, or wrestler. It ultimately derives from the name of the Parthians, called the *Pahlav* in the Middle Persian of the Sasanian period and *Pahla* during the Islamic period. This is the name used by the last ruling family of Iran, the Pahlavi dynasty of the 20th century. The word *pahlavān* was transmitted to India during the Mughal period and became *pahalwān* ("wrestler"), a word used universally across the subcontinent today.

"I am both wolf and helper." Dēnkard 8.16.26.13

Javānmardi has a more ancient root. The origin lies in the Avestan *mairyō* – the wolf warriors of the oldest layer of Iranian history. This became *marīka* ("warrior") in Old Persian, in turn becoming the Middle Persian word *mard-juwān* ("young man").

Eventually the institution of *javānmardi* (literally "principles of young men") emerged. The *Šahnāme* extolls the virtues of *javānmardi*. This pre-Islamic set of rules for *javānmardān* ("young knights") influenced the Arabic concept of *futuwwa* ("young-manliness"), and is related to European chivalry.

From the outset, the Iranian spirit fostered the creation of elite warrior bands. The "Immortals" of the Achaemenid dynasty were the 10,000 strong bodyguard of the king deployed where the fighting was fiercest. According to the Greek historian Hēródotos, they were said to be immortal because if one died in battle, he was replaced so there were always exactly 10,000 members.

Achaemenid Persian nobles were given a rigorous military training in youth in companies of fifty. They were taught to run, swim, ride horses, shoot, stand watch, and march long distance; at twenty years old, they entered the military for around thirty years. It was these men who made up the Immortals of Darius and Xerxes. The later Sasanian dynasty resurrected the Immortals until they fell to the Arabic forces in the 7th century CE. The final emergence of the elite Immortals was under the last two shahs of Iran who utilised the *Gārd-e Jāvidān* ("Immortal Guard").

"This indeed is my activity: inasmuch as my body has the strength, as battle-fighter I am a good battle fighter... Trained am I both with hands and with feet. As a horseman I am a good horseman. As a bowman I am a good bowman both afoot and on horseback. As a spearman I am a good spearman both afoot and on horseback." Inscription B of Darius I at Naqš-e Rostam

Javānmardi is also known as *'Ayyārī*. *'Ayyārān* ("helpers") were confraternal organisations ruled by *javānmardi*. These "scoundrels," as they were also known, were descended from Sasanian *asbarān* ("horsemen") – elite cavalry units of independent means. Aristocratic men of the Sasanian period aspired to be *asbarān*, whose social standards were shaped into ethical and moral standards called *āzādegi* ("free-spiritedness").

Ayyārān groups, some of which were bandits and brigands, had initiation ceremonies for new members to ensure they were a *javānmard*. The Arabic *futuwwa* initiation included the "ritual of the cup," in which the initiate would drink the "Wine of Malakut." This vow of commitment is rooted in the *haoma* ritual of Zoroastrianism and echoed in Roman Mithraism, where the *krater* ("cup") was employed. The grail mythos of the European knights also stems from the same roots.

"In the estimation of the wise, the world is a false gem that passes each moment from one hand to another." Sa'dī Shīrāzī, Būstān

In the 9th century CE, a coppersmith by the name of Laith wrote a moral guide for his sons. One of these sons was to become Yaʿqub ibn al-Laith al-Saffār, founder of the Iranian Saffarid dynasty that ruled from 861 until 1003. Laith set out seven principles: follow the way of manliness (*javānmardi*), be honest and tell the truth at all times, keep secrets, show magnanimity towards friends and enemies, safeguard material goods that are entrusted into your care, keep promises, and "honour the salt" (if you share food with someone, you are bound to them).

These principles of Laith are a form of the ideal classical sense of *javānmardi*. A *javānmard* is a noble man with a sense of identity. He keeps his word and speaks the truth. He is pure in word, thought, and deed. He always perseveres and is valorous, avoiding harming the innocent and standing up against tyrannical cruelty as a champion of these who cannot fight for themselves.

He contents himself with modest profit in business, preferring to lose his property rather than benefit from another's misfortune. He is trustworthy, generous, humble, honest, and sincere. He shuns envy and hypocrisy.

He is gentle in speech and makes a special effort to help friends and relatives. He strives to maintain his reputation, valuing honour, integrity, gratitude, and directness. He gives without being asked and lives without fear.

Assassins

"The whole universe is made rational and familiar; so that no helplessness is felt before the most awesome attempt at orientation; men are to be grown up and at home beyond all horizons. To be an Ismāʿīlī is to be of the elite of the universe."
Marshall Hodgson, The Secret Order of the Assassins

The elite warrior band spirit of Iran reared its head again in the 11th century during the occupation of Iran by the Saljūq Turks. In 1090, the militant Nizārī Ismāʿīlī Iranian Hasan-i Sabbāh captured the castle of Alamūt in the Alborz mountains north of Tehran.

Hasan-i Sabbāh was the first of eight lords who ruled from Alamūt ("Eagle's Nest") between 1090 and 1256. The "Old Man of the Mountain" and his "Assassins" waged guerrilla war on the Saljūqs for almost two hundred years.

Hasan-i Sabbāh was born in the Iranian city of Qom, to a Twelver Shīʿa family. However, after a journey of religious discovery, became an Ismāʿīlī. Returning to Iran from Egypt, which was ruled by the Ismāʿīlī Fatimid dynasty, Sabbāh gathered his forces and took Alamūt.

From 1090 until his death in 1124, Hasan remained in his house on Alamūt. He left only twice in the 34 years of his rule. It was from this building that he planned, wrote, and directed operations against the Saljūqs.

> *"The doubt he feels is precisely the rising to consciousness and the exteriorisation of the Darkness which had remained hidden within him, and which from then on he can conquer and hurl outside of himself."* Henry Corbin, Cyclical Time and Ismāʿīlī Gnosis

He sent his daughters and their mother away, beginning the precedent that Ismāʿīlī chieftains never had their womenfolk with them while executing a military command. In his severity, he executed his own sons for breaking his laws. He possessed intense, severe logic.

Hasan was also grounded in a will toward attaining and embodying a universal doctrine of truth. This *hudad*, or anthropocentrism, is the Assassin doctrine of representing Cosmic principles through the microcosm of man.

Nizārī Ismāʿīlīs see the human form as perfect. All things must pass through human form before they can attain spiritual perfection.

In turn, the Ismāʿīlīs have a tripartite division of men. The *ālē tedād* are the ignorant common masses who require Sharīʿa (Islamic law). The *xvās* are the elite capable of esoteric understanding through the *taʾlim* ("instruction") of an *Imām*, who puts them on the *ṭarīqa* (spiritual path). The *axas-ī xvās* are the super elite who recognise the ultimate nature of reality through *taʾyid* (direct inspiration).

The Assassins were the elite *mojāhedīn* (holy warriors) who fought from deep within occupied territory. They were also an initiatory order with degrees of spiritual initiation. They fought both the lesser and Greater Holy War while guided by the principles of Nizārī Ismāʿīlīsm and *javānmardi*. Following the sacking of Alamūt and the end of the Assassins, Ismāʿīlīs in Iran went underground, assimilating into Ṣufīsm, adding their mysticism to the movement.

Luṭis

"You have hard work ahead of you, and those you confront will sometimes be wolves, sometimes sheep." Šahnāme

With roots in the *ʿayyār* and *Ṣufī* brotherhoods, the *luṭis* came to prominence in the 19th century. Belonging to the lower social classes, *luṭis* aimed at embodying *javānmardi*. They held that the noble traits were not limited to higher social classes. Instead, these could be cultivated by any man who led the appropriate lifestyle and behaved according to the precepts of *javānmardi*, which was also known as *luṭigari*.

Luṭis were often employed as fruit and drink peddlers, working on the streets of their neighbourhoods. They had a strong camaraderie and dressed in a distinctive manner, wearing emblems of their membership. These seven items were a chain from Yazd, a brass bowl from Kermān, a silk handkerchief from Kāšān, a knife from Eṣfahān, a cherry wood pipe, a shawl, and cotton slippers.

"I should gain a reputation as long as there is death. If I die with a good name, that is good." Šarif Muḥammad

These initially itinerant men were at first looked upon poorly by society; but by the 19th century, they had reputations as guardians of the streets they patrolled. The *luṭis* were seen as Robin Hood-type bandits, making them the spiritual successors to the *'ayyārān*. The term initially denoted a "bandit" or "vagabond," but they began to be known as *luṭi-ye ḵodāʾi* ("godly *luṭi*") and *luṭi-ye allāhi* ("*luṭi* devoted to God") as their reputations improved.

They were strongmen, often performing feats of athleticism and strength for the benefit of their community. They had to abide by the rules of *javānmardi*, which earned them the respect of the local people. They became associated with the neighbourhood *zurxāne*, and until the 20th century the membership of these houses of strength was mostly made up of *luṭis*. They were known for their friendly wrestling bouts in the *zurxāne* and fights to defend their honour on the streets against *penti* ("thugs").

"He whose strength does not suffice to drive away the evil desires that tempt him, that man does not even reach the rank of beasts." Ibn Sīnā (Avicenna), Recital of the Bird

Because of their fighting skills, the *luṭis* were eventually used by the 19th century Qajar dynasty governmental and religious organisations as enforcers and protection detail. By the 20th century they were often subverted to act as professional protesters and thugs, becoming increasingly volatile, chaotic, and violent. Both Shah Mohammad Reza Pahlavi and the Islamic Revolutionary forces employed *luṭis* in the late 1970s, with many of them forming the backbone of the *Basij*, a paramilitary auxiliary volunteer force that forms part of the Iranian Revolutionary Guard.

Pahlavānān

"His heart was wise, his mind prudent; his shoulders were those of a warrior, his mind that of a priest." Šahnāme

Pahlavānān ("champions") are men who train in the *zurxāne*. Originally the term *pahlavān* – which came to be associated with *koštigir* ("wrestler") – designated a fully proficient warrior. These warriors trained in the martial art of *varzeš-e pahlavāni* ("heroic sport") at the *zurxāne*.

Maintaining both a physical prowess and a chivalrous code, the *pahlavānān* represent all that is noble about the Iranian spirit. They have always stood up for the good. They continued to preserve the fire of the moral Indo-European wolf warrior, even when forced to take it underground while ruled by outside forces.

While maintaining *javānmardi*, *pahlavānān* trace their origins back to the Indo-Iranian period. The structure of the training regimen itself can be seen in the Achaemenid training of the nobles. They woke at dawn, prayed for strength of mind and body, and then practiced their physical exercises.

To this day, *pahlavānān* wake early, even though the modern *zurxāne* changed the training time from morning to evening. Pahlavān Xorāsāni introduced night training in the 20th century. They maintain an early awakening like their ancestors did to emulate Mithra, who is "ever wakeful" and the "enemy of sloth."

"Vitality and strength are what I wish to attend me." Yasna 43.1

The *pahlavān* is courageous, strong, capable, helpful, honest, and an enemy of falsehood. He is imbued with *āzādegi* ("free-spiritedness"), a sign of his strength. The concept that physical wellbeing goes hand-in-hand with moral welfare is an ancient Iranian concept and the *haurvatāt* ("wholeness"), and *amərətatāt* ("immortality") of the Zarathuštrian doctrine is evidenced in the ageless strength, good health, and freedom from sickness espoused in the *zurxāne*.

Due to the *pahlavānān*, Iran has retained its sovereignty over the millennia despite foreign invasions. When the Mongols and the Saljūq Turks banned the Iranians from training with weapons, they went underground into the cave-like *zurxāne* where they continued to practice archery and swordsmanship in secret. After the Iranians took back their country, the shahs retained *pahlavānān* for their entertainment as wrestlers, but also for protection. *Pahlavānān* would patrol and guard the city at night during the Safavid period, much like the *luṭis* of the Qajar times.

"Ride hard. Shoot straight. Speak the truth." Ancient Iranian saying

The *pahlavān* is historically expected to emulate Rostam, being able to cross mountains and deserts, assail fortresses, and be able to use any weapon. He must be pure of spirit and stout of heart; he must be righteous in thought, word, and deed. He must be chivalrous, humble and polite, with a love of his people and a sense of duty towards them. The *pahlavānān* practice charitable giving to the unfortunate in their community, distributing donations from wealthy patrons of the *zurxāne* to the poor.

The *pahlavān* must love life, Light, and God. Aside from Rostam, the *pahlavān* particularly seek to emulate Imām ʿAlī, who is viewed as the first *javānmard*. The call of his name echoes through the *zurxāne* throughout the *varzeš-e pahlavāni* practice.

The level to which these tenets are put into practice is rarely seen in the modern world. The *pahlavānān* of Iran genuinely and zealously take these qualities to heart, earnestly practicing them. They are not just lofty ideals, but practically implemented behaviours that are found in members of any *zurxāne* anywhere in the country.

Similar to a fraternity, they form a brotherhood of men who look after each other and have an obligation to ensure each member stays true to the morality of *pahlavāni*. Magnanimous in victory, they are careful not to cause humiliation to others, avoiding making their opponent look weak in the eyes of observers. They are welcoming and generous to strangers, while keeping a vigilant eye over them.

"He attained exaltation by his perfection. He dispelled darkness with his beauty." **Sa'dī Shīrāzī, Golestān**

The WarYogin embodies the spirit of *javānmardi* and *pahlavāni*. He stands upright among the ruins of the modern world, refusing to stoop and become corrupted by the material plane. He is pure and righteous. He is vigilant over his body and mind.

The WarYogin seeks the higher plane so that he may be more effective in the physical world. He is a beacon of light that radiates out into the gloom that surrounds him. Casting out his positive aura into the world, he remains true to what is always true, to universal cosmic order.

While doing so, he does not tread on others in order to ascend. He stands against the forces of Darkness not only for himself, but for the world. He is the defender of what is good; he is both wolf and helper.

"Fight only with opposing warriors; harm no one who offers you no harm." **Šahnāme**

Zurxāne

"Our house of sport is not the place for the lascivious. This place is for the pure, this house is not for the unpurified. Oh my heart, stay in this house of strength for a while. Find a way in the ruins and religious hymns." Masnavi-ye Gokošti-ye Mirnejāt

The *zurxāne* is a "house of strength." There, *pahlavānān* practice the ancient ritual of strength known as *varzeš-e pahlavāni* ("heroic sport"). Sometimes called *varzeš-e bastani* ("ancient sport"), athletes train in physical practices geared towards fighting, and utilise training tools that emulate weapons of war.

The *zurxāne* has always been a place of strength and moral education. It was known in ancient times as a *langargāh* ("anchorage") or *āmājxāne* ("House of Shooting").

From the late middle ages until the mid-20th century, the *zurxāne* was associated primarily with wrestling. They were almost identical to the wrestlers' *tekke*s (Persian *takia* – "lodges") of Ottoman Turkey, *harkara*s of Afghanistan, and *akhara*s of India. They are privately owned, but open to the public. Some of the buildings are over 500 years old and still in use to this day.

Almost every traditional neighbourhood has a *zurxāne*. Found in the back alleys of cities, they are almost invisible from the outside. They have an unassuming, almost unnoticeable exterior. Only a small sign usually announces that it is a *zurxāne*.

The *zurxāne* has a small door so that everyone who enters, regardless of station in life, must bow and show humility and modesty to enter. Shoes must be removed at the door. A narrow corridor then leads to an expansive domed inner chamber reminiscent of the Mithraic cave of initiation or a Ṣufī lodge.

"Then strike with all your strength at the door of God; destroy the mountain of the self." Farīd ud-Dīn 'Aṭṭār, Conference of the Birds

The traditional *zurxāne* is architecturally similar to the public bathhouse, and many traditional bathhouses were connected to *zurxāne*, sometimes having one in their compound. The main room of the *zurxāne* is sunken slightly below street level to ensure a constant temperature, and prevent drafts that might harm perspiring athletes. The high domed roof has windows for light to come in; the high ceiling reverberates the sounds of the *zarb* (drum), *zang* (bell), and chanting that accompany the training. This creates a highly charged spiritual atmosphere.

In the centre of the room is the *go'd* ("hollow" or "deep"), a sunken pit that is either hexagonal, octagonal, square, or round. The *go'd* is a sacred space in which activities of the *zurxāne* take place. The hexagonal *go'd* is a reference to the tomb of Imām ʿAlī, which originally had six sides. The octagonal go'd represents the eighth *Imām*, Imām Reza (Alī ibn Mūsā al-Riḍā). The original shape for a *go'd* is circular, sometimes called the "circle of love."

The folkloric origin of the *go'd* is said to lie in the custom of two warring factions choosing one champion each to represent their side. A pit would be dug, and the two opposing champions would fight to the death in proxy of a full-scale battle. The dead man would then be buried in the pit.

"There is no escape from the death we are born to, and the world is nothing but a cradle for the grave." Šahnāme

The width of the *go'd* varies greatly, but newer *zurxāne* tend to have wider ones with a diameter of around thirty-three feet. The *go'd* is low to remind the *pahlavānān* to remain humble. It is approximately three feet deep.

The surface was originally made of brushwood and ash covered in a layer of clay and earth. This was moistened with water every day, providing a soft surface for wrestling. The modern *go'd* is usually made of wood or stone and covered with linoleum, carpet, or wrestling mats.

The *go'd* faces the *sardam*, an elevated platform near the entrance of the *zurxāne* which has a staircase leading up to it. The *sardam* is the seat of the *moršed* ("master" or "guide"), who plays the drum and bell while chanting *masnavī* (poetry) by Persian masters like Saʿdī, Ḥāfeẓ,

Rūmī, and Ferdowsī. Only the *moršed* may enter the *sardam* as it is a sacred place. The walls of the *sardam* and all around the *zurxāne* are adorned with pictures of athletes and saints, as well as verses from holy scripture.

Around the *go'd* is a flat surface to accommodate additional practitioners and equipment, as well as seating for spectators. The highest seating is for the most important visitor. In the past this was next to the *sardam*, but in modern practice it is now on the opposite side, facing the *sardam*. Everyone is expected to give up their seat to whoever is older or more senior than him.

"Humility is the only ritual for a devotee. If you desire greatness, be humble; no other ladder is there by which to climb." Sa'dī Shīrāzī, Būstān

Javānmardi is practiced in the *zurxāne*. Regardless of a man's status outside of the *zurxāne*, inside everyone is viewed as an equal. The *pahlavān* puts on the *tombān* (wrestling pants) or *long* (sarong-style cloth), joining his noble comrades in performing his physical and spiritual exercises.

It is said "the spirit of Rostam can be found in the *zurxāne*." In the *Šahnāme*, Kay Kāvus places his son Siyāvaš in Rostam's care of so he can be trained in the arts of fighting and *javānmardi*. The *zurxāne's* aim is to create ideal warriors and enemies of falsehood: valiant, capable, powerful, honourable *pahlavān*. The *zurxāne* fosters sportsmanship, modesty, humbleness, and altruism, shunning arrogance, envy, lust, and pride. It is where men strive toward the divine realm.

This is done through the practice of *varzeš-e pahlavāni* ("heroic sport"). It is sometimes known by the misnomer *varzeš-e bastani* ("ancient sport") due to the foundation of the Federation of Ancient Athletics in the 1950s by the last Shah of Iran. Prior to that time, the term had never been used.

Varzeš-e pahlavāni is a system of physical and spiritual training developed over thousands of years. The roots lie in the ancient Iranian martial arts, with tools and exercises designed to prepare the *pahlavān* for battle. The physical aims are to build strength, endurance, stamina, agility, speed, flexibility, and concentration.

"From warriors learn courage, and wisdom from the sage. If you truly seek God's grace, ride with the heavenly carriage."
Šams-od-Dīn Ḥāfeẓ-e Šīrāzī, Rubaiyat 23

Varzeš-e pahlavāni was born from warfare. At its heart are the needs of warriors who had to engage in hand-to-hand combat. It is focussed on making fearless fighters who are capable whether armed with the spear, mace and sword, or disarmed among a horde of enemies.

Varzeš-e pahlavāni aims to forge warriors of men. It does so by preparing them for the battlefield of life. In order to achieve this, body, mind, and spirit must be trained to razor sharp perfection.

Varzeš-e pahlavāni promotes ethical and moral values. It imbues a respect for order and truth. It creates a warrior who is humble, generous, brave, and virtuous. It makes men who are able to safeguard the local community, as well as the nation and its traditions.

Material gain has never had a place in *varzeš-e pahlavāni*. Trophies, medals, and prizes have never been sought out. An example of this is the famous wrestler Gholamreza Takhti, who on several occasions proved that honour was more important to him than victory. In his match against Soviet wrestler Aleksandr Medved, he refused to attack Medved's injured leg, leading to a loss. The *bazuband* (champion's armlet), historically awarded to the *jahān pahlavān* ("world champion"), in Iran has always been a symbol of *javānmardi*, not only wrestling skill.

"Make the spirit of wisdom a protection for the back, and wear the spirit of contentment on the body, like arms and armour and valour, and make the spirit of truth a shield, the spirit of thankfulness a club, the spirit of complete mindfulness a bow, and the spirit of liberality an arrow; and they make the spirit of moderation like a spear, the spirit of perseverance a gauntlet, and then put forth the spirit of destiny as a protection." Dādestān-ī Mēnōg-ī Xrad 43.6-13

The traditions of the *zurxāne* have developed over the millennia with influences from across the Iranian diaspora. Various Iranian schools of thought and religious practices have had their impact on the *zurxāne* from Mithraism and Zoroastrianism, to Islam, and Ṣufīsm.

The name *zurxāne* was not known before the Islamic period, but some scholars have placed its origins in the Mithraic initiatory caves. Notable Iranologist and Persian mythologist Mehrdād Bahār connected the *pahlavānān* and *zurxāne* to Mithraism. He demonstrated how the *zurxāne* is a cave-like underground fraternity governed by a code of ethics in the vein of the pre-Islamic Mithraic brotherhoods, who also cultivated physical, mental, and spiritual abilities.

In his book *Tarikh-e Iran-e Bastan* (History of Ancient Iran), Iranian Prime Minister and scholar Hassan Pirnia connected the word *pahlavān* to *Pahlav* ("Parthian"). Pirnia also posited that the *Šahnāme* of Ferdowsī drew from the Parthian heroes and their practices. The Parthians were Mithraists, and the religion peaked during their reign. They came into direct contact with the Romans, clashing with them across the buffer territory of Armenia and bringing their religion to the Europeans. Members of the Roman cult of Mithras were almost entirely soldiers, as were the Parthian Mithraic warriors from whom they took their religion. This militaristic streak connects them to the *pahlavānān* of the *zurxāne*.

"We worship Mithra… whom the warriors worship at the manes of their horses, requesting strength for their teams, health for themselves." Mihr Yašt 10.10-11

Proponents of Mithraic origins cite an overall similarity of the *zurxāne* and Mithraic temples that emerged in the Roman era, since like the other Iranians, the Parthians worshipped Mithra on mountain peaks. Both *zurxāne* and Mithraic temples are underground and close to a source of water. Some scholars say the ringing of a bell originates in the revealing of the image of the sun at the end of Mithraic ceremony, and that chanting reflects the recitation of hymns to Mithra.

The strict hierarchies within the *zurxāne* are said to reflect the seven grades of Mithraic initiation. The exclusion of women from *zurxāne* is also said to originate from Mithraic ritual rather than Islam. This reflects how Mithraism was in essence a religion for warrior elite.

While there is a connection to Mithraism, it is more likely a cultural one rather than direct correlation. Certain elements of the *zurxāne* tradition can be acknowledged to derive from Mithraic warrior practices, but the *Mithraea-zurxāne* conflation is a more tenuous theory.

The word *zurxāne* does not appear until the Islamic period, which correlates to training in the fighting arts going underground during the 7th century Arab invasion of Iran. Even after their conversion to Islam, Arab governors forbade the training in weapons of their Iranian subjects. This is likely what brought about the *zurxāne* as it is known today.

"It is the sacred duty of the highest culture to maintain the strongest battalions." Ernst Jünger, *War as an Inner Experience*

It is likely the *zurxāne* originated with 8th century chieftains of Xorāsān province in Eastern Iran, the Sistān of Rostam and *Airyanəm Vaējah* ("Expanse of the Aryans") of Zarathuštra. Descended from the

Parthians and led by a man named Ustadh Sis, these warrior elites rebelled against the Abbasid Caliphate in 767. Since they were forbidden to train, the rebels used cellars and other underground locations to prepare for their short-lived uprising.

The first recorded building of a *zurxāne* for the specific purpose of training *varzeš-e pahlavāni* is in the 13th or 14th century. It was constructed by a famous *pahlavān* called Puryā-ye Vali (Pahlavān Mahmud al-Khwārizmī) from Xwārazm in what is now Uzbekistan and Turkmenistan. Likewise, the exercises of the *zurxāne* are first described in the Safavid-era *Scroll of Puryā-ye Vali*.

Puryā-ye Vali is considered the archetypical *pahlavān*. His poetry is still recited in the *zurxāne*.

The first European account of the *zurxāne* was written by Sir John Chardin, a 17th century French aristocrat and traveller. His book, *The Travels of Sir John Chardin in Persia* (see Appendix I), has a short vignette of the *zurxāne*. However, he only discusses wrestling without commenting on the other equipment.

"They call the Place where they Show themselves to Wrestle, Zour Kone, that is to say, The House of Force. They have of 'em in all the Houses of their great Lords, and especially of the Governours of Provinces, to Exercise their People. Every Town has besides Companies of those Wrestlers for show." Sir John Chardin, Travels in Persia

The next European account of the *zurxāne* describes a scene much closer in comparison to the modern iteration. Carsten Niebuhr, a German explorer in the employ of the Danish court visited a *zurxāne* in the 1760s. In his book *Account of Travels to Arabia and Other Surrounding Lands* (see Appendix II) he depicts a high-ceilinged, semi-subterranean room where the *pahlavānān* are performing exercises that can be recognised today. As the weapons of war changed, the need to practice archery and other traditional weapon craft diminished. Instead, *varzeš-e pahlavāni* developed into a more stylised system of practice with symbolic weaponry as the training tools.

Under the rule of the Turkic Qājār dynasty, the *zurxāne* thrived. The Qājār rulers were enthusiastic patrons of wrestling and funded the construction of new *zurxāne*. Nāser-ad-Din Šāh-e Qājār (reigned 1848-1896) in particular built many *zurxāne*, bringing *varzeš-e pahlavāni* to its peak of popularity. It was during Qājār rule that the *luṭis* became a prominent component of the *pahlavānān* community. Men of higher status often built their own *zurxāne* so they could train privately without the lower-class element.

"At Shiraz there are three such public Surchône, where not only persons of the middle and lower rank, but sometimes also noble military and civil servants, gather to strengthen their bodies by such exercises. The great gentlemen sometimes have rooms in their houses set up for this purpose, in order to wrestle there with their friends and acquaintances." **Carsten Niebuhr, Account of travels to Arabia and other surrounding lands**

After the Constitutional Revolution of 1905, royal patronage ended, leading to a diminishing of the sport. The upper classes abandoned the *zurxāne*, leaving it to the lower and middle strata of society. By the 1920s, western sports and modern entertainment further hit the popularity of the *zurxāne*, sending it into a terminal decline.

As the state took over the role of policing neighbourhoods, the need for local men to protect their community was reduced, hitting the *zurxāne* again. *Varzeš-e pahlavāni* was kept alive by a small, dedicated group of amateurs with help from some of the members of the Iranian elite who founded the *Jam'iyat-e gordān-e Irān* ("Society of Iranian Heroes") in 1924 to preserve the tradition and make it respectable. It was in this period that training shifted from a morning, to an evening practice.

All this was happening against a barrage of negative propaganda from the Iranian press, who relentlessly attacked the *zurxāne* as being a corrupt, unhygienic, and outdated institution filled with thugs: a remnant of the disliked Qājār dynasty. The press claimed that it no longer met the modern needs of Iran and pushed instead for Western sports and training methods. Despite this, the *zurxāne* survived, and just as its days looked numbered it was thrown a lifeline in 1934.

In that year, the thousandth anniversary of the birth of the poet Ferdowsī was celebrated. Exhibitions of *varzeš-e pahlavāni*, then called *varzeš-e qadim* ("old sport"), was made a part of the program for nationwide celebrations, bringing it back to the fore once again. The Twelver Shī'a elements that had permeated the sport from early

Islamic times were emphasised, making the sport appear morally and culturally more relevant to the Iranian government.

"I escaped from the fourteen coffins and the ten tombs from which emanated the shadow of God so that I would be taken towards the sacred world." Šehāb-al-dīn Yaḥyā Sohravardī, The Recital of the Occidental Exile

In 1934, then crown prince, Mohammad Reza Pahlavi made *varzeš-e pahlavāni* exhibitions part of his wedding celebration. The future shah was keen to bring Iran back to its ancient roots, in particular the glory of the Achaemenid dynasty. He renamed the sport *varzeš-e bāstāni* (ancient sport) for his wedding to imply a pre-Islamic origin.

This coincided with a renewed interest in *javānmardi*, thanks in part to Moḥammad-Tāqi Bahār (poet laureate of Iran) writing a series of articles in the 1940s. These linked *javānmardi* specifically to the *zurxāne* tradition. He particularly highlighted the patriotic nature of the early days of the *zurxāne*, making it highly esteemed in the public eye once again.

By the 1960s, the popularity of the *zurxāne* once more waned, with many private facilities closing. Some were taken over by the state or large corporations, but many vanished.

After the Islamic Revolution in 1978-79, the government began to revive the tradition once again, emphasising the Islamic nature of the *zurxāne* and permitting young boys (who were previously excluded) from participating. In the past, only men who could grow beards were allowed to train. *Pahlavānān* were required to wear t-shirts to preserve their modesty in line with the law. Previously, they had always been bare-chested (often tattooed), to signify the equalising nature of being in the *zurxāne*.

"Spirits are corporealised and bodies spiritualised. Through and in the world, ways of being and moral behaviour are personalised, and super sensory realities are manifested in the forms and figures with which they symbolise." Muḥsin Fayẓ Kāšānī, Hidden Words

The modern practice of *varzeš-e pahlavāni* has been consolidated and regulated with competitions requiring standard methods and exercises. The International Zurkhaneh Sport Federation in Tehran is the official governing body. Due to various internal disputes however, Mašhad in Xorāsān-e Razavi province has become the de facto capital of *varzeš-e pahlavāni* under the patronage of the Āstān-e Qods-e Razavi trust.

There are currently around five hundred *zurxāne* in Iran, but the tradition is once more losing popularity. Younger generations are more interested in the trappings of modern life and western sports. In this era of general dissolution, it is more important than ever for the sacred militant spirit to keep the *zurxāne* alive. The *zurxāne* has survived waves of foreign invasion from Arabs, Turks, and Mongols.

A new generation need to take up the banner and fight for what matters, for what has always been important. The Indo-European martial tradition of Iran is the training ground of holy warriors. The WarYogin must take his place among the champions to ensure the *zurxāne* can be passed on to future generations of heroes.

"If a man leaves behind him a noble reputation, he should not despair when he has to depart." Šahnāme

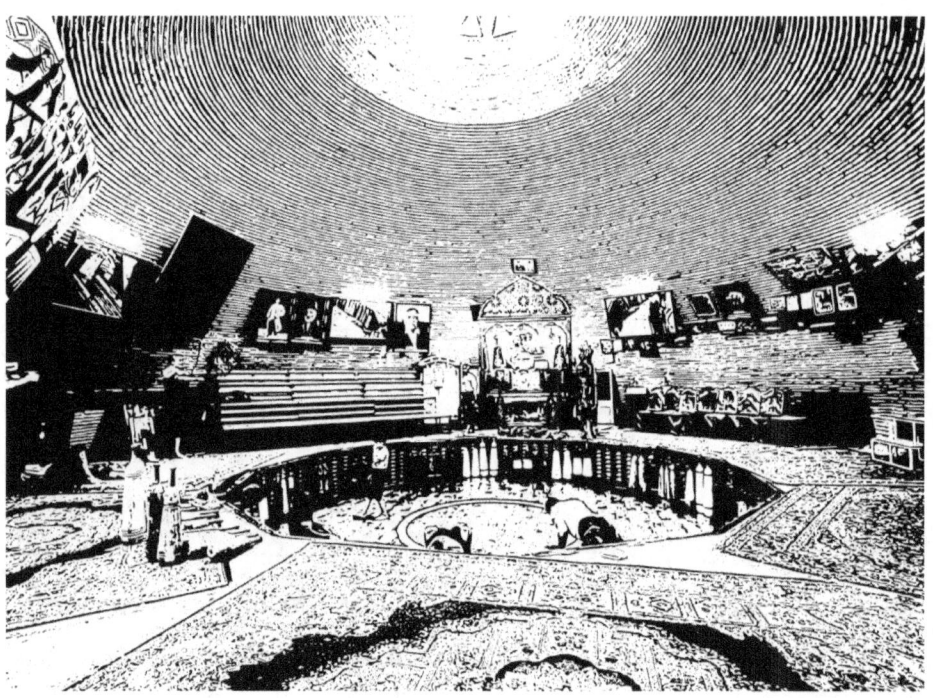

Hierarchy

"A man with merit is he who observes good toil through merit, through conference and deliberation and power and wisdom after good toil he considers much, keeps the name away from idleness, in order to attain greatness and worthiness through wisdom and character." Him vā Kherat ī Farkho Gabra 2

A man's social status in public life has no bearing of his ranking within the *zurxāne*. This was traditionally denoted by training barechested. The only matter that determines merit and superiority is experience. This is an iron-clad structure that cannot be violated. A veteran *pahlavān* does not defer to a novice or lower ranked athlete at any point, regardless of his standing outside the *zurxāne*.

Aside from the ranking, there are some specialist positions such as the *moršed* ("guide") who sings and plays the music to lead the exercises, and the *xādem* ("servant") who acts as a caretaker and looks after the needs of the *pahlavānān*. All members, including the *moršed* and *xādem* are able to perform the exercises. The *moršed* and *xādem* are usually experienced athletes who have a long association with the *zurxāne*. Some *zurxāne* also have a *moštemālči* ("masseur"), but this is not common.

In addition to these roles, the other important figure is the *miyāndār* ("leader") who stands in the centre of the *go'd* leading the exercises. This is not necessarily one man's job, and the *miyāndār* may change depending on the exercise being performed. It is always a senior *pahlavān* who acts as *miyāndār*.

> *"Since I have been a warrior I have lifted my head as high as the sun."* Šahnāme

The *moršed* is the highest position within the *zurxāne*. He harmonises the athlete's moves and chants words of wisdom to educate the athletes and remind them of the virtues of heroes. In the ancient past he was a trumpeter, a drill master, or a standard bearer.

The *moršed* must be skilled in all the exercises of *varzeš-e pahlavāni*, as well as having cultivated a strong spiritual level. In addition, he must know all of the songs and chants used during practice. He must be able to sing while he plays the goblet-shaped *zarb* ("drum") and inverted bowl-shaped *zang* ("bell"), both of which give a martial atmosphere. It is the most important role and must be fulfilled by a highly capable individual.

The *moršed* employs his exceptional understanding to keep the pace of the exercises while being responsive to what is happening in the *go'd*. Using the *homayun* musical mode, he must pick the right verse and rhythm for any situation from a vast canon of spiritual and poetic works. This includes the *Šahnāme*, *Qoran*, poems praising Imām ʿAlī, and works by famous Iranian poets.

The *moršed* is responsible for the spiritual, moral, and religious education of the *pahlavānān*. He enables them to partake in the Ṣufī practice of sama ("listening"). This involves the recitation of poetry or music.

"Ours is the method of alchemy, it involves extracting the subtle organism of light from beneath the mountains under which it lies imprisoned." Najm ad-Dīn al-Kobrā, The Blossoms of Beauty and the Perfumes of Majesty 12

The *moršed* is also the master of ceremonies, acknowledging senior members with the drum, bell, and a chant as they enter the *zurxāne*. For example, when an experienced athlete enters, the *moršed* calls out "Welcome!" Athletes then chant a *salavāt* (divine blessings on Muḥammad), in his honour: "God bless Muḥammad and his family!" When a veteran enters, the *moršed* calls out "your arrival is most prosperous and delightful" before everyone chants a *salavāt*.

The *miyāndār* (known as a *kohnesavār*, or "senior rider" in the past) is the *pahlavān* who leads the exercises from the centre of the *go'd*. As such, he must be highly skilled.

The *miyāndār* is drawn from the *sādāt* (literally "descendents of the Prophet"); these are senior members of the *zurxāne*. He is responsible for keeping the pace within the *go'd* and communicating with the *moršed* on both a verbal and non-verbal level, as well as demonstrating correct technique to the novices.

Using visual and verbal cues, the *moršed* and *miyāndār* control the pace and transitions between exercises. The role of *miyāndār* may shift depending on who is the best at a particular exercise. The *moršed* and *miyāndār* lead the prayers and *salavāt* which punctuate the entire practice.

"No one can reach there or force a passage save the Elect among the mass of men, those who have gained a strength that does not originally belong to man by right." Ibn Sīnā (Avicenna), Recital of Ḥayy ibn Yaqẓān 10

The ranking in the *zurxāne* is referred to as *kesvat* ("merit"). The only merit is experience and there is no fast track to higher ranks. Neither is there testing, nor any kind of marker of rank to denote who is who.

The position the *pahlavān* takes in the *go'd* is the only outward sign of his standing. The lowest ranked members are at the "bottom" of the *go'd* facing the *sardam*, while the higher ranks stand at the "top", directly in front and facing away from the *sardam*. Visiting athletes are accorded the highest respect and given a high position in the *go'd* in front of the *sardam*. *Kesvat* is not based on practical experience alone, but also takes strength, technical ability, age, spiritual maturity, and reputation into account.

"The north quarter of the world is your dwelling place." Mahmūd Šabestarī, Rose Garden of Secrets

In the past, there were several grades of athlete, each wearing the *long* (sarong-style cloth) in a different manner. From the mid-20th century, this disappeared and the standard ranks were put in place. In ascending order, they are *noče* ("novice"), *noxāste* ("beginner"), and *pahlavān* ("champion").

Traditionally, it took two years for a newcomer to attain the rank of a *noče*. After ten years, the athlete was socially accepted and approved by the elders. Some athletes wear the *long*, but most wear the *tombān-e nataʾi* (shortened to *tombān*) or *šalvār-e košti*: the leather or cloth wrestling pants embroidered with highly decorative designs. The choice of *tombān* does not denote rank.

Above the standard *pahlavān* are the *sādāt* (singular *sayed*), or elders. *Sayed* denotes a descendent of the Prophet Muḥammad, which can be both literal and figurative. A *sayed* is honoured above all others. When calling out to the athletes to acclaim their skill, the *moršed* will say different phrases based on their rank. For example, a skilled athlete will be saluted with "Māshāʾallāh!" ("God has willed it!"). A veteran may be saluted as "Rostam, the iron man from Zābol!"

"Of all realities that man sees and contemplates in the world beyond, those which delight… as well as their opposites… none of these is extrinsic to him, to the very essence of his soul, none is distinct or separate from his own act of existing." Ṣadr ad-Dīn Muḥammad Šīrāzī (Mullā Ṣadra), Book of the Theosophy of the Throne

The highest rank for merit is *jahān pahlavān* ("world champion"), an honour given out at the annual wrestling tournament. This is also a reference to Rostam, who is given the title "Champion of All the World" by Kavus. The champion's armband awarded to the *jahān pahlavān* is the clasp of Rostam. Aside from world champion, there are several champion grades for state sponsored wrestlers and Olympic champions.

Within the *zurxāne*, these are all classified as senior members. Entering the *go'd* is done in order of seniority from highest to lowest, as are the exercises. *Taxte-ye šeno* (push-up boards) and *mil* (wooden clubs) are picked up by the oldest first. Other exercises are done by the youngest first. This strict order is part of the moral education that makes the *zurxāne* the heart of the social structure of a warrior society.

"God's glory is with me; I am both prince and priest. I hold evil doers back from their evil and I guide souls towards the light." Šahnāme

Entering the Go'd

"I swam in the primordial and ultimate oceans, in eternity and subsistence, and I discovered the unveiling of the Essence and Attributes which deaf stones and lofty mountains cannot endure." Rūzbihān Baqlī, **Unveiling of Secrets**

After the *pahlavānān* have put on their *long* or *tombān*, they line up to enter the *go'd*. Just as ablution must be performed before prayer, athletes must be washed and clean before entering the *go'd*, as it is a sacred space. *Pahlavānān* enter the *go'd* in order of seniority, with guests being accorded the highest honour.

After the *moršed* has taken his place in the *sardam*, he begins to play. The *miyāndār* or senior athlete raises his right hand and calls out *roxat* ("permission"). The *moršed* answers *forsat* ("chance"). All athletes must ask permission from the *moršed* in order to enter the *go'd*. *Roxat* is called out by athletes before every individual exercise, as well as by the *miyāndār* before leading each exercise.

The athlete steps into the *go'd* with his right foot first and exits with his left foot first. This is because the right is considered pure while the left is less so. Stepping into the sacred space should be done with the purer side and vice versa.

After descending the steps into the *go'd*, each athlete bends one knee, touches the floor with the two fingers of his right hand, kisses them, and touches his forehead. This act, called *zamīn buse* ("kiss the earth") is said to be a tribute to the famous *pahlavān* Puryā-ye Vali, but may have deeper roots. In ancient times, the heroes would bend down and kiss the ground to acknowledge that they came from the earth, and upon death they would return to it.

"First, one should respect the kohnesavār (miyāndār) more than one's own father. Because if he does not respect the kohnesavār he will not reach the highest level of goodness and will die in his youth." Scroll of Puryā-ye Vali

The *moršed* plays a rhythm that the athletes enter to. They march around in a slow and rhythmic motion with footwork known as *pāy-e šāteri* ("camel steps"), circling the *go'd* as everyone enters in turn. The *miyāndār* leads this march around the *go'd*, which is sometimes called the *šelangandazi* ("hose laying").

The arms are swung from side to side. While doing this, the feet march with the heels raised high towards the buttocks in turn. It is a way of limbering up prior to exercise. This is performed while everyone enters the *go'd*.

Once everyone has entered the *go'd*, the athletes circle and warm up. This lasts until they reach their designated positions with a *taxte-ye šeno* ("push-up board"). The highest ranked and visiting athletes are directly under the *sardam* with their backs to the *moršed*.

Conversely, the novices are on the far side of the *go'd* facing the *moršed*. This placement is not just a matter of respect for the *moršed*, but also a practical matter. The less-experienced athletes can see what the *moršed* is doing and benefit from his direct supervision.

"On the meridian line he stands upright, casting no shadow before or behind, on the right hand or on the left." Mahmūd Šhabestarī, Rose Garden of Secrets

The *go'd* represents a place outside of profane time and space. That which is outside of the *go'd* and *sardam* are detached from the sacred enclosure. The athletes enter a timeless realm where they perform a powerful warrior ritual.

The *go'd* is low, reminding them of their vows of humility, as well as rooting them in the fertile ancestral soil. The *sardam* is high, causing the athletes to look upward to the celestial. It is decorated with peacock and dove feathers that adorned battle helmets in ancient times. Shaped like a triumphal arch, the *sardam* spurs the heroes to strive for victory against both external and internal opponents.

In the *go'd*, the *pahlavānān* must be clean, bare-footed, and appropriately dressed. Originally they were bare-chested to signify the irrelevance of external hierarchies. Fooling around, swearing, badmouthing and speaking behind others' backs, smoking, and consuming intoxicants is forbidden in the *zurxāne* and absolutely unthinkable in the *go'd* itself.

While in the *go'd*, everyone must obey the *miyāndār* who occupies the central position while the others are in a circle around him. The *miyāndār* asks permission from the *moršed* before taking his position in the centre. The *miyāndār* offers his role to other experienced athletes before accepting, though everyone refuses to take his place.

The *miyāndār* follows the *moršed*'s rhythm. The athletes follow the *miyāndār*. No athlete may do an exercise that the *miyāndār* is not performing, nor may he stand idle. Nobody may speak while the *miyāndār* is speaking or praying, and all require his permission to leave the *go'd*.

"As long as your essence is realised within you in a constant state, you are you forever, while with this body, you are not." Šehāb-al-dīn Yaḥyā Sohravardī, The Shape of Light

The *garm kardan* (warm up) is the first activity that commences within the *go'd*. This starts with the marching in a circle as everyone enters. Sometimes various arm movements will be done to limber up while this circling of the *go'd* takes place.

The *miyāndār* then takes his *taxte-ye šeno* from the stack at the side of the *go'd* without breaking his stride. He picks it up from the

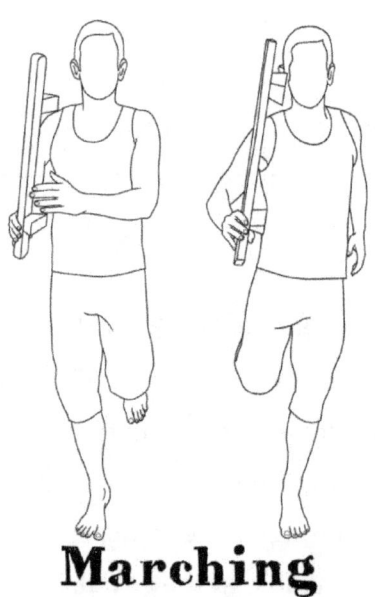

Marching with Taxte

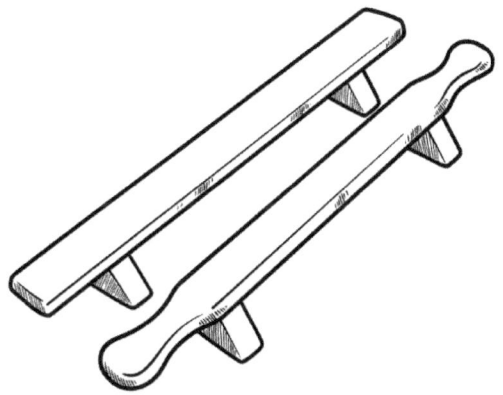 centre with his right hand; then using his left hand, he transfers his grip to the bottom of the *taxte*, holding it like a sword. The other athletes all follow suit in order of seniority.

The *taxte* is a rectangular wooden board that is 4 inches wide, 32 inches long, and stands on two trapezoidal feet that are 2 inches high. Some have sword handle shaped ends as a nod to the *šamšir* ("sword") it is modelled from. Athletes may kiss the *taxte* as a sign of respect.

They continue the march as when they first entered the *go'd* until the *miyāndār* stops in the highest position and asks permission to lead. He then heads to the centre and everyone places their *taxte* in front of them horizontally. All of the athletes take up the *konde zadan* ("kneeling") position, also known as the *salam zurxāne* ("*zurxāne* greeting"), or the *salam bastani* ("ancient greeting"), behind their *taxte*.

The left foot is planted on the floor with the right knee on the ground. The left hand is placed on the left knee and the right hand on the right hip. This is an ancient position signifying the respect held by a *pahlavān* to the highest authority while still able to jump into action swiftly if required.

Old men are allowed to place both knees on top of the *taxte* with their feet behind them. The feet are never placed on the *taxte*, as this is a sign of disrespect. All athletes remain in this attentive position while the *moršed* performs the *fātiḥ bismillāh* (opening prayer), sings a song, or recites a poem. Then the *pahlavānān* stand and prepare for the *šeno* exercises.

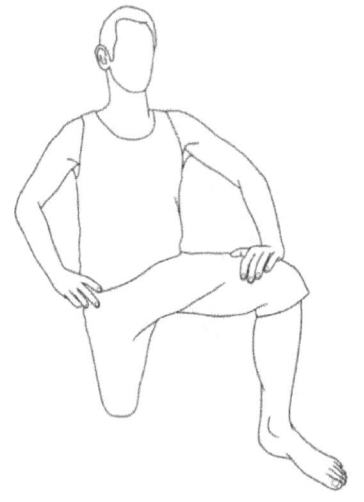

Konde Zadan

"The essence of the unrighteous will be the worst, but the righteous will have the best." Yasna 30.4

Šeno

"One should do the push-ups no more than one hundred times because otherwise it will be harmful. The principle of doing push-ups is that one rests upon both palms of the hands and tiptoes, and the knees and belly should not touch the ground." Scroll of Puryā-ye Vali

One of the most iconic sets of exercises in *varzeš-e pahlavāni* is the *šeno* sequence. These are push-up exercises that use the *taxte-ye šeno*. There is a dispute as to whether the term *šenā* or *šeno* should be used. *Šenā* means "swim," but this is not a particularly accurate description of the motion used for the exercise. *Šeno* is derived from the word *šenoftan* ("listen") and makes sense once you consider the context of the use of the *taxte-ye šeno*.

The push-up was originally performed by soldiers in the field using their *šamšir* (sword) as a base on sandy ground. This is why the *pā baz* (wide-legged stance) also developed. The element of "listening" comes from placing the ear against the ground to listen for enemies intent on battle.

After the *moršed* has concluded his opening ritual, the *šeno raftan* ("performance of *šeno*") begins. With the music of the *moršed*

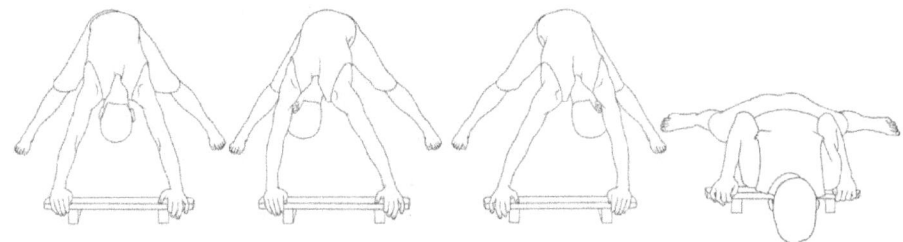

Šeno-ye Sarnavāzi

determining the rhythm, the *miyāndār* leads athletes through the first sequence of push-ups. The initial sequence is called *šeno-ye sarnavāzi* ("head *šeno*"), known as "four-count split push-ups" in the West.

With the hands placed on each side of the top of the *taxte*, the hips are raised into an "inverted V" position. The feet are spread wide apart with the feet flat on the floor. From this position, on the first count the whole body is lowered so that the *taxte* touches the chest, the torso is horizontal, and the feet make contact with the ground on their inner side.

The body is then returned to the starting position on the second count. The body is softened and the head is nodded to the right on the third count. It is then nodded to the left on the fourth count, before starting the whole sequence again. This is done in time with all of the athletes in the *go'd* with the *miyāndār* leading.

"I, O Zarathuštra, am righteous Haoma who keeps death away. Seek me, O Spitamid; press me out for drinking; praise me for strength as future Saošyants will praise me." Hōm Yašt, Yasna 9.2

After a number of these have been done for several minutes, the *miyāndār* calls out "ʿAlī!" to indicate a pace change into the second sequence of *šeno*. This is the *šeno-ye šallāghi* ("whipping *šeno*"), known in the West as the "two-count split push-up." It is the same as the *sarnavāzi*, except it has no third and fourth count with the head motion. Instead, it is a simple up into the first position and down into the second position for several minutes and plenty of repetitions.

The athletes either rest over their *taxte* in a neutral position while still holding the board, or they stand up. Here the *miyāndār* and *moršed* may interact with some inspirational words or prayers. This short break precedes the third sequence called the *šeno-ye pājoft* ("feet-together *šeno*"). With the hands on the same *taxte* position, the feet are placed together with the legs in contact with each other.

First, following the call of *yek* ("one") by the *miyāndār*, a single push-up is performed before returning to the inverted V position, followed by a few seconds rest. Next, on the call of *do* ("two"), two

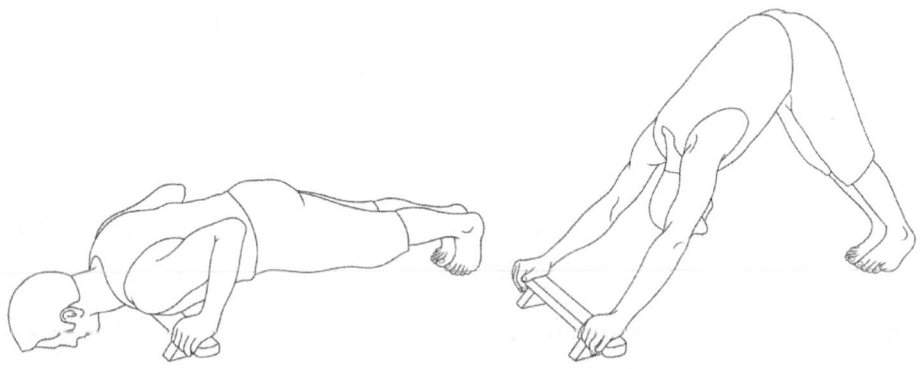

Šeno-ye Pājoft

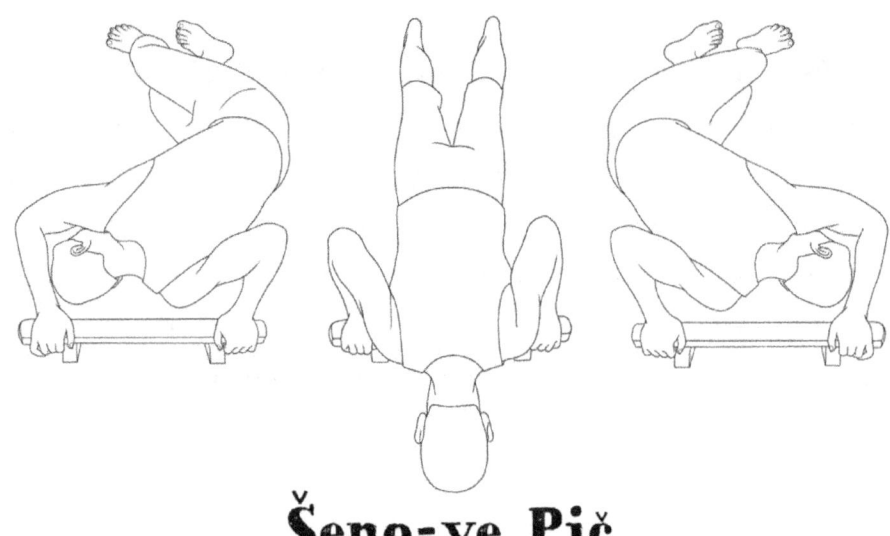

Šeno-ye Pič

push-ups are performed back-to-back with a few seconds rest. Then, on the call of *se* ("three"), three push-ups are performed back-to-back.

Finally, the *miyāndār* calls out "ʿAlī!" to indicate the final phase of the *pājoft*. A single push-up is performed, then the athlete returns to the inverted V position. The right heel is pushed to the ground, followed by the left in a pedalling motion to make a four-count, much like with the head in the *sarnavāzi*. This is repeated until the *miyāndār* signals to the *moršed* that the athletes have done enough.

"Brave men seek results with a sword." Šahnāme

Following the *pājoft*, the final push up exercise is performed. The *šeno-ye pič* ("spiral *šeno*"), known in the West as a "crescent moon push-up," starts with the chest touching the *taxte* in a plank position, with the feet slightly apart. The right elbow raises and the body curls, putting the head under the right arm.

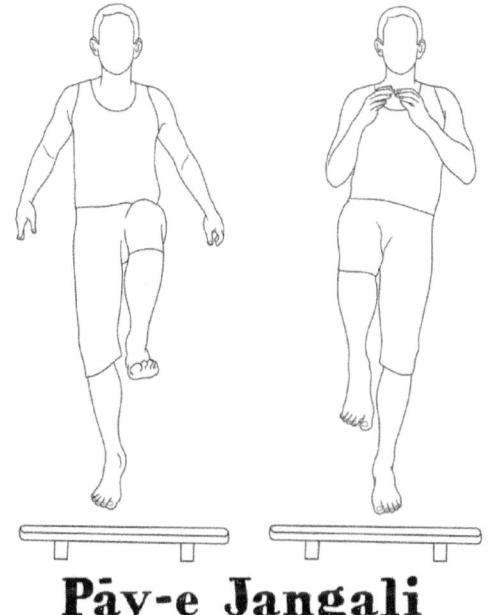

Pāy-e Jangali

The feet turn at the same time as the body curl, allowing the inside of the right foot and the outside of the left foot to touch the ground. This is all done without allowing the hips to rise from the low plank position. The body returns to the starting position and then mirrors the motion on the left side, transitioning smoothly from side to side until the *miyāndār* is done.

At this point everyone stands up behind their *taxte* and begins to perform marching steps called *pāy-e jangali* ("jungle steps"), or *pāy-e pošte taxte* ("steps behind the *taxte*"). The knees are raised high at the front in turn, in a jumping, marching motion. Both arms are swung back simultaneously while the left knee is lifted up and swung forward when the right knee is lifted up.

At this point, the *miyāndār* and possibly some other athletes may hold the *taxte* like a sword and perform sword slashes and strikes in the air.

The *miyāndār* then exits the centre with his *taxte*, rejoining the circle. He then asks again for permission from the seniors before retaking the centre position, or he gives it up for another to take the role of *miyāndār* for the next phase of the *zurxāne* ritual. The entire *šeno* phase of exercise lasts around ten to fifteen minutes.

"We called you, but you did not migrate. We indicated to you, but you did not understand... if you wish to deliver yourself and your brother, do not hold yourself back from your decision to travel." Šehāb-al-dīn Yaḥyā Sohravardī, The Recital of the Occidental Exile

Narmeš and Xamgiri

"Fate has brought you up for this day. In this battle against Ahriman you must not rest." Šahnāme

Narmeš, or *narm kardan*, are stretches for mobility of the upper body. They are performed behind the *taxte-ye šeno*, followed by *xamgiri* (leg stretches and squats), in preparation for swinging the *mil* (wooden clubs), and as a way of recovering after the *šeno* exercises. These stretches are performed one after the other with fluid transitions that are marked by the *miyāndār's* verbal and non-verbal cues. He also calls out "ʿAlī!" for any change of pace to a more "heroic" level of exercise.

The duration of the entire phase is between five and ten minutes.

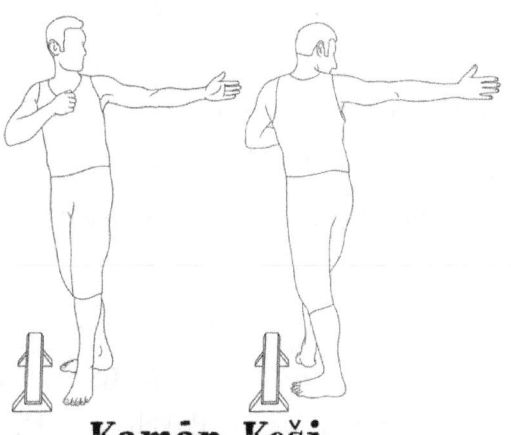
Kamān Keši

The first exercise performed is the *kamān keši* ("draw the bow"). Standing upright, with the feet a little closer than shoulder-width apart, the torso is turned to the right. This is performed

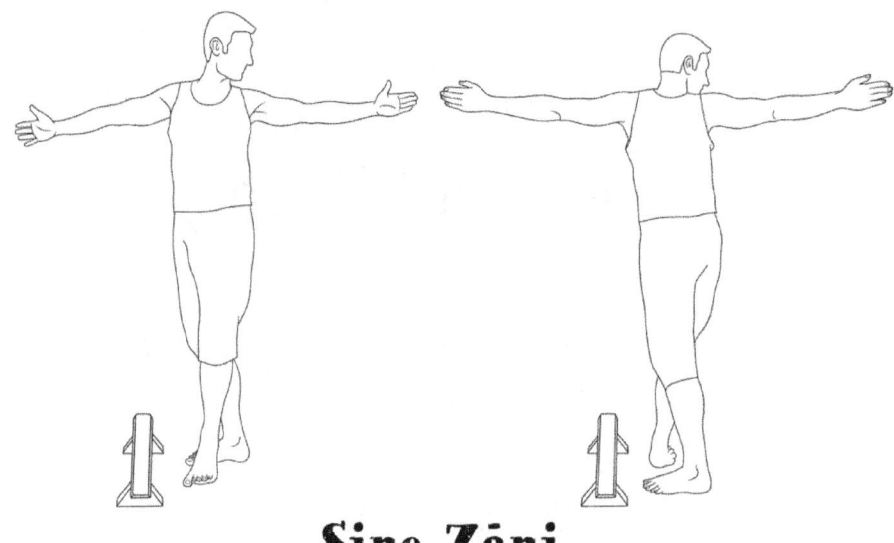

Sine Zāni

with the right arm extended to the side and the left hand at the chest with the elbow extended to the left, as though one were drawing a bow back.

To facilitate the turn, the right foot is allowed to pivot slightly. From here, the torso is turned the other way with the hands switching position in the middle of the turn, so that the left becomes the extended arm and the right hand is at the chest. This should be performed rhythmically and with an expansion of the chest.

"Your essence, your rational soul, is not material, nor does it relate to matter. It is from time and space; therefore it cannot be perceived by the senses." Šehāb-al-dīn Yaḥyā Sohravardī, The Shape of Light

After several repetitions, the *miyāndār* calls out "ʿAlī!" to signify the transition to the next exercise: *sine zāni* ("hitting the chest"). This

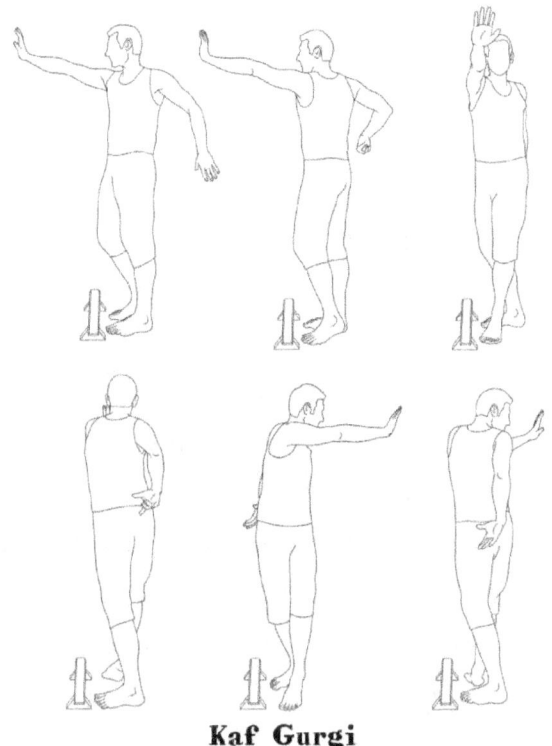
Kaf Gurgi

is similar to *kamān keši*, except both hands are extended at the twist of the torso. At the transition point, both hands touch the chest before opening again for the twist on the other side.

Next is *kaf gurgi* ("wolf slap"). With the feet in the same position as before, the torso is twisted while the right hand is pushed forward and the arm extended at the front. The left arm is allowed to be relaxed, but trailed behind. The hands touch the centre of the chest at the frontal transition point, before the left hand is pushed forward with the right trailing behind.

The next transition of this same move (after several repetitions) pushes the right hand out to the left side, then the left hand to the right, giving a deeper twist to the torso. Finally, the third stage of *kaf gurgi* is to turn the body almost completely pushing the right arm straight out behind and to the left and vice versa. The feet are turned to enable this, with the left foot pivoting as the right arm is extended behind; then the right foot is turned with the left hand extended.

> "He scattered his enemies like a wolf." Šahnāme

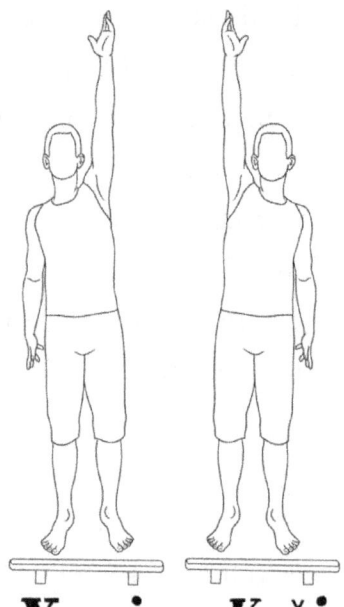

Xanjar Keši

The next stretch is *xanjar keši* ("draw the dagger"). The feet remain in place. The right hand swings up in front of the body in a straight line from the shoulder to reach up above the head. The left hand reaches downwards by the left leg. At this point, the feet should be on tip toes. The feet drop to being flat as the hands swing up and down respectively to switch, so that the left is reaching upwards and the right is by the side of the thigh.

After several repetitions, this transitions to *zanjir zani* ("whip with the scourge"). Rotating to the right, both arms are raised upwards above the head. The feet are used to pivot and allow for a perpendicular turn. The body is then turned to the other side with the arms dropping down at the centre point and swinging upward again on the other side. After several repetitions of this, two arm raises are done on each side before turning. Finally, three raises are done on each side without turning.

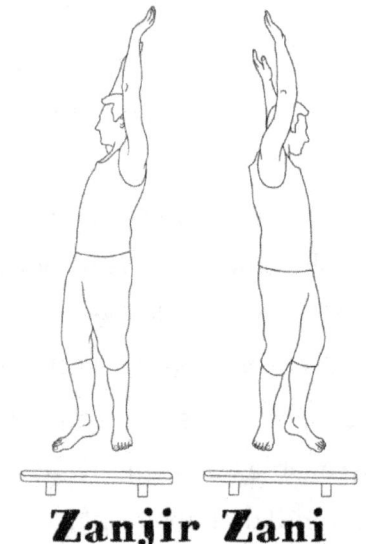

Zanjir Zani

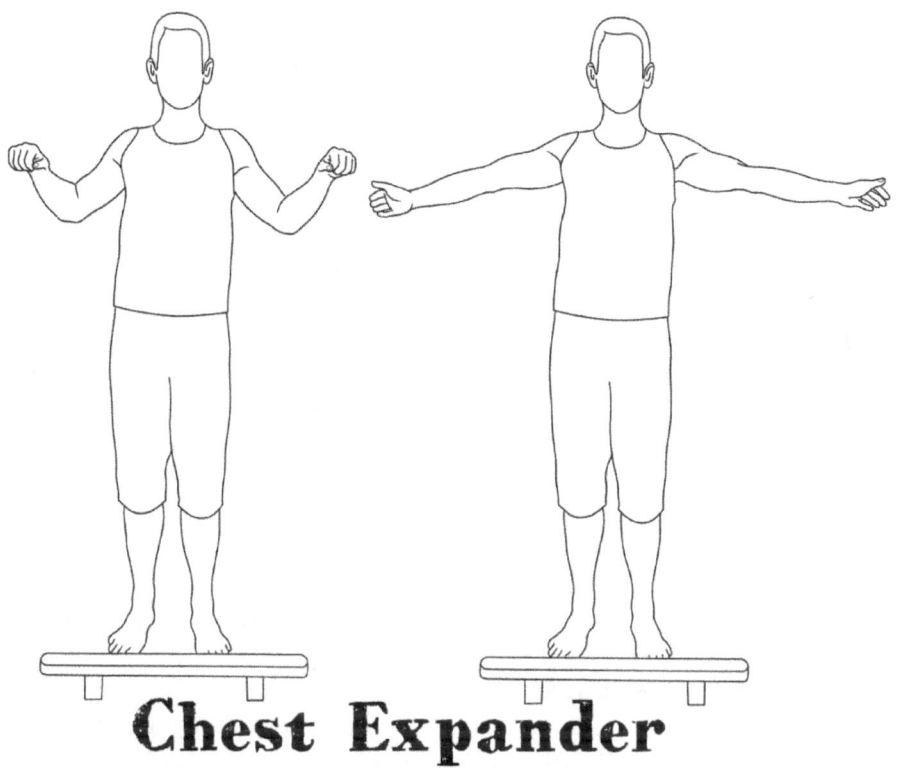

Chest Expander

"His entrancing state is the union of union, His heart ravishing beauty the light of light." Mahmūd Šubestarī, Rose Garden of Secrets

Next, a nameless chest expander is done, much like the common iteration. The hands are brought together with the arms extended directly in front of the chest, the arms are bent, and the elbows are sent backwards to open the chest. Then after returning to the front position, the fully extended arms are sent backwards on the same trajectory. Alternating between bent and extended arms, this is repeated several times.

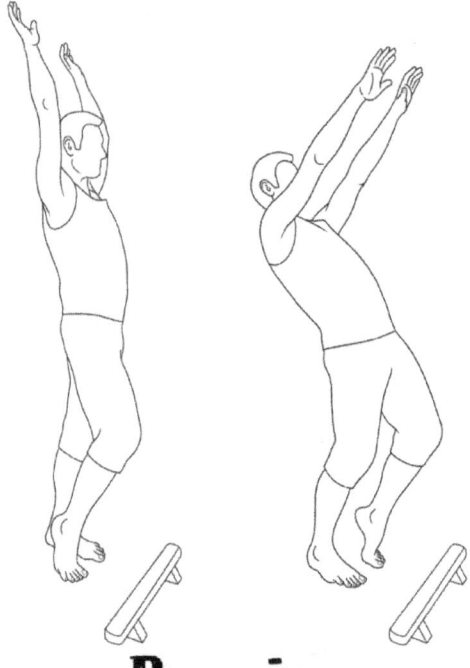

Parvāne

Following on from this is *parvāne* ("butterfly"). The arms are swung from the centre, down to the sides, arching upwards as the shoulders lean back. The left knee is bent forward while the right leg remains straight. The hands come together at the top in this position.

The body returns to the neutral position with the arms returning on the same trajectory. They are then lifted straight up in front of the body until they are above the head. The right knee bends while the body remains straight.

"O menial, vigorously make you known of what sort I am, and of what sort my skilfulnesses, and of what sort my superiority." Inscription B of Darius I at Naqš-e Rostam

Following this is *salib* ("cross"), which is initially done to a four-second four count. Marching on the spot, the arms are raised up above the head on the one count. The hands then touch the shoulders twice with the elbows out to the sides to the two count. The arms are then extended out into a cross shape on the three count; finally, they are brought down to the sides on the four count.

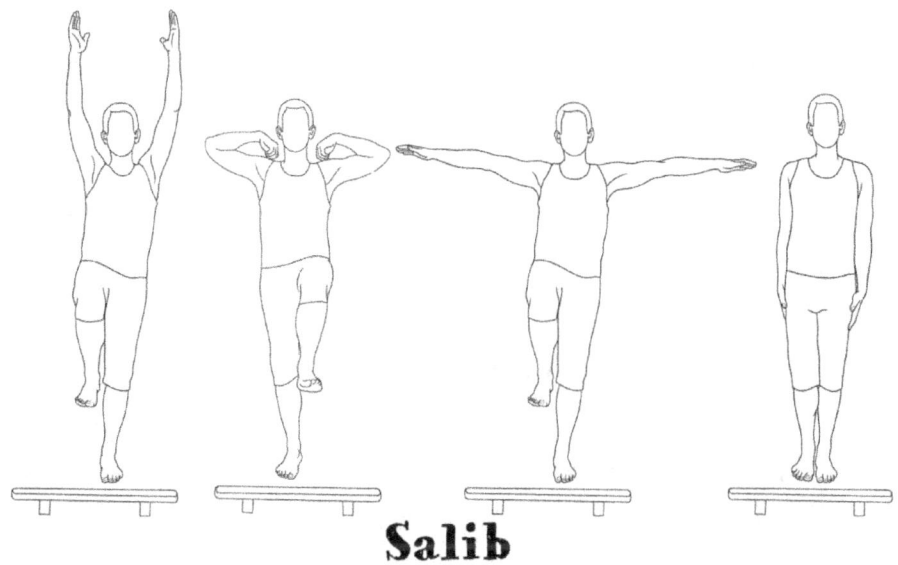

Salib

After a number of repetitions, the speed is increased to a two-second four count. Instead of marching both feet are jumped on the spot on each arm motion.

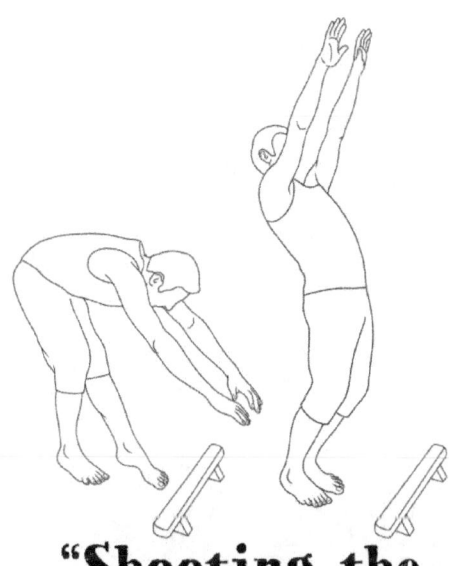

"Shooting the Single Leg"

The *salib* is the last exercise of the *narmeš* section. Seamlessly following on is the *xamgiri* ("leg moves") part of the practice. The first exercise of this part is also called *xamgiri* but is explained as "shooting the single leg."

Hinging forward at the waist, the right leg is bent with the foot flat on the floor, while the left leg is pointed out with a slight bend in front of the body. The ball of the left foot remains in contact with the ground. As this is done, the arms are brought together in a grabbing motion just above the left knee.

The legs return to neutral standing as the arms arch back the way they came, but continuing their trajectory to arch together over the head as the chest leans back a little. The downward motion is repeated, this time with the left leg bent and the right extended.

"God is beautiful and He loves beauty." Al-Mu'jam al-Awsat 6906

After several repetitions, the same exercise is performed. This time however, at the bottom it is doubled up with the left foot forward, then the right foot forward and the grabbing motion on each before coming up to the top position. Then, after several repetitions,

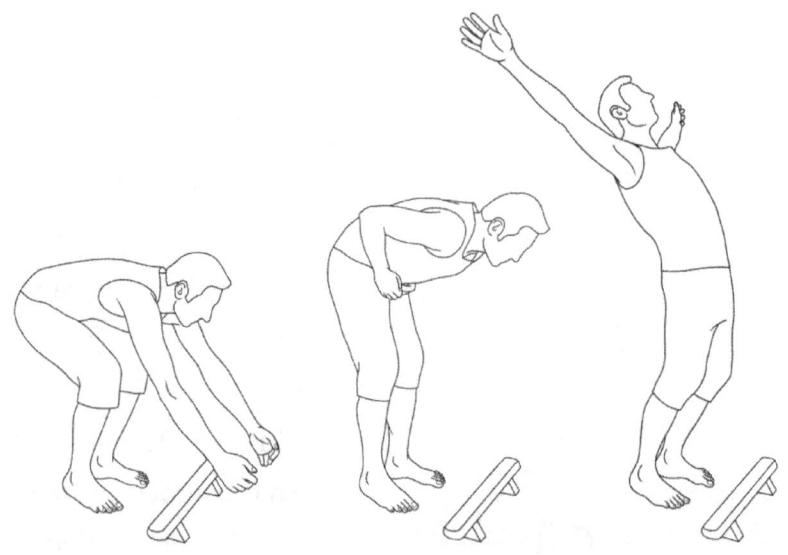

Xamir Giri

the bottom end footwork is done three times: left, right, and then both legs are bent together.

The next leg exercise is *xamir giri* ("kneading the dough"). The body is hinged at the waist and the knees of both legs are bent; the hands extend out below the knees and pull upwards to the stomach area as though one were kneading dough. This is done with a small bounce in the motion three times, before standing upright and arching the arms to the sides and upwards above the head. This is followed by a low jump before being performed again.

"The kingly soul lays waste the body, and after its destruction he builds it anew." Jalāl al-Dīn Muḥammad Rūmī, Masnavi 1.2

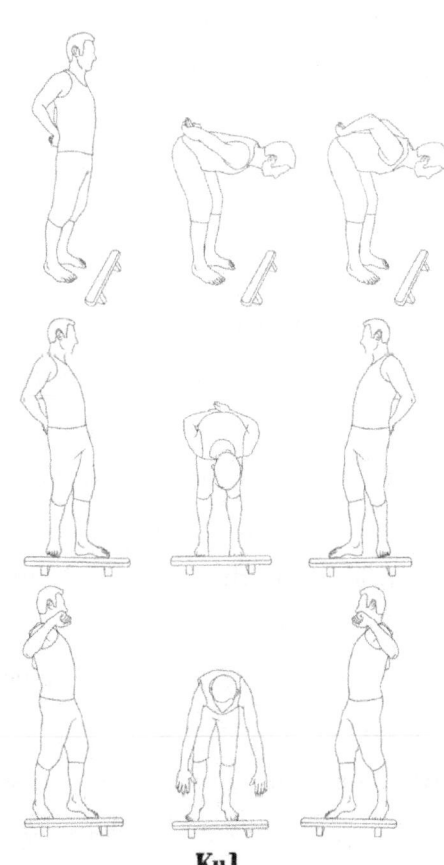

Kul

An exercise known as *kul* (muscle shaping) follows. The hands are clasped at the small of the back and the torso hinges at the waist. The torso is lifted slightly up and down while the shoulders are rolled back three times. Standing straight up, the elbows are quickly popped backwards while the hands

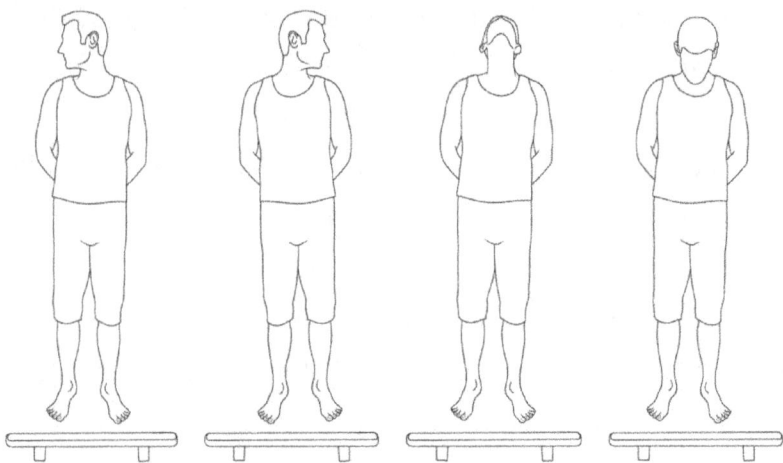

Narbiši Gardan

remain clasped. This is repeated a few times, before the exercise changes to a rotational movement.

Facing right with the feet pivoted, the elbows are popped back before the body is turned while hinging at the waist, then returning to an upright position facing left and popping the elbows again. This transitions into a third phase where the hands are released and swing with the rotation to a bent arm chest expansion on each side.

After this is *narbiši gardan* ("neck shaping"). With the hands behind the back, the head is rotated side-to-side for several repetitions and then up and down for several more.

The final exercise of the *xamgiri* section is *nešastan va barxāstan* ("sitting and standing"). The feet are placed a little wider than shoulder-width apart. The arms move forward to the sides in a grabbing motion as the legs squat. Standing up, the right foot is stepped back, followed by the left. The right is stepped forward, followed by the left, followed by a squat.

After performing this with single squats for a number of repetitions, it is then done with two squats before stepping forward and back. Then it is done with three squats. After the call of "ʿAlī!" the squat is performed without the steps until the *moršed* stops the beat of the drum.

"May we be among those who bring about the transfiguration of the earth" Yasna 30.9

When the *miyāndār* picks up his *taxte* like a sword, everyone follows suit and all march vigorously on the spot in the *pāy-e šāteri* ("messenger steps"). Here, the *miyāndār* may slash and thrust the *taxte* as a sword, or simply keep the rhythm with the rest of the athletes. The *taxte* are then returned to their storage in order of seniority.

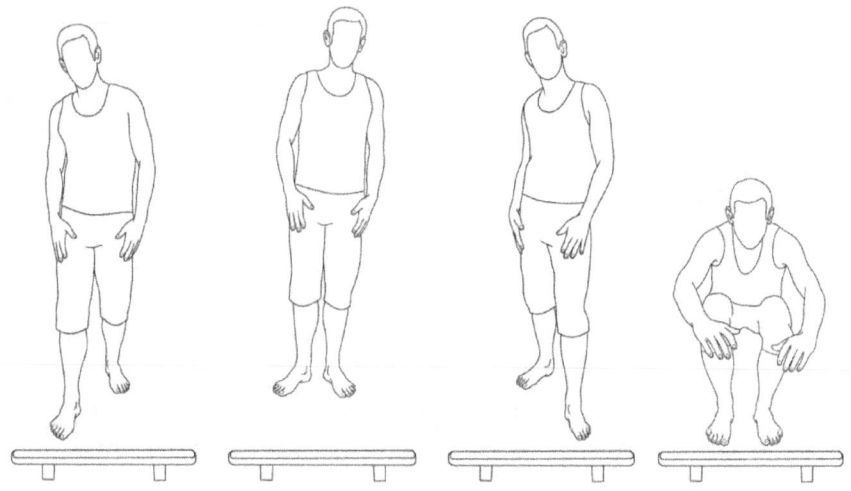

Nešastan Va Barxâstan

"Do not make light of any enemy, no matter how unworthy he may be." Šahnāme

Mil

"The benefit of taking mil is... he can pull at the thigh of the opponent easily and throw him above the head." Tumār-e Puryā-ye Vali

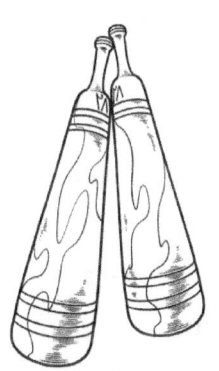

After the *taxte-ye šeno* have been put back, the *pahlavānān* take a pair of *mil* ("pillar") each in order of seniority and return to their positions. *Mil* are conical-shaped wooden clubs that vary in weight from 7 lbs each upwards, and are traditionally fashioned from walnut, elm, argan, or ash. Many light *mil* are made of pine also. They are measured as pairs, so a 14 lb pair are 7 lbs each.

During the main practice, most athletes work with light *mil* – normally a 22 lb pair. Light mil are more common as the old saying goes: *"If you want your body to be strong, practice with heavy sang and light mil."*

Heavy *mil* swings, with pairs of up to 140 lbs are performed by *mil* specialists who compete to see who can swing the heaviest set. The *mil* are swung one after the other in a four-count and a two-count.

They symbolise the battlefield mace and shield, with one swung over the shoulder while the other is held in a shield position, mimicking the technique used in war.

There is much debate on the grip that the *mil* are held with. The "pinkie grip" involves the little finger being placed under the pommel, while the standard grip has the little finger with the others above the pommel. Proponents of the pinkie grip say that it allows for a deeper front position and therefore a deeper stretch and range of motion. However, the standard grip allows for both of these also, since the hand is relaxed at the front of the swing and tightened at the back. Since it is a simulated battlefield weapon, a standard grip would be more useful, as it gives more control over the *mil* in general.

Heavy mil must be swung with a standard grip, as the pinkie grip does not give enough control at higher weights. The official line of the International Zurkhaneh Sports Federation is that a standard grip must be employed in competition. The Iranian national champions all use a standard grip as the consensus among them is that the pinkie grip places the delicate bones of the hand in a compromised position.

"We worship Mithra… who grasps in both hands the mace with a hundred knobs, with a hundred blades, a feller of men as it swings forward, cast in strong golden bronze, the strongest of weapons, the most victorious of weapons." Mihr Yašt 10.96

After the athletes are in position with the *mil* stood up in front of them, the *miyāndār* takes up his *mil* followed by the rest of the men in the *go'd*. The *mil* are swung out directly in front of the body and arced up to the shoulders, with the hands low by the waist and the wide head of the *mil* resting on the shoulders in preparation for the *milgiri* ("*mil* moves") or *milvarzi* ("*mil* work").

To the rhythm of the *moršed*, they begin the *gavorgeh* (four-count swings). *Gavorgeh* ("tip of wrist") is a loan word from Mongolian, and sometimes the term *sar moč* ("head wrist") is used. The right *mil* is raised and swung over the shoulder and behind the head (not over the head) as the right foot steps to the right and the left foot is pivoted and slid towards the right, initiating a 45 degree turn to the left as the *mil* is swung on the right side.

When the *mil* is behind the back, the hand holding it should be low on the nape of the neck and the bicep should brush the ear. The *mil* is controlled throughout the swing until it returns to its position in front of the right shoulder with the hand loose on the handle by the hip. The left is then swung in the same manner, with the left foot stepping and the right sliding and pivoting to turn the body to the other side.

The feet are kept closer than shoulder-width apart throughout. The head of the *mil* may make contact with the shoulder at the front or may be kept an inch or so away for a no-touch style. The *gavorgeh* is done to a four-count with each side being two counts.

"The Promethean element obeys the individual soul, and never bows to collective rule. Hence soul must find the way of Return." Henry Corbin, Avicenna and the Visionary Recital

During the *gavorgeh* phase, the *miyāndār* (and anyone else with enough room to do so) may perform *širin kari* ("sweet work"). These are fancy swings of various kings including outward swings, levers, downwards swings, and so on. They are a way for the *pahlavān* to revel in his skill and show what he is capable of as an individual among the collective. In *varzeš-e pahlavāni* competition, the team may perform *širin kari* in order to distinguish themselves from the others.

After the *gavorgeh* swings, the *mil* are put down on the floor in front of the athlete while the *miyāndār* and *moršed* offer up a prayer. Once the *mil* are placed back on the floor, the athletes perform a *mil xamgiri*. With both hands placed on the top of the pommels of each *mil*, the body is hinged down at the waist while tipping the right *mil* as a lever to the floor and keeping the left *mil* upright with the hand still on the pommel.

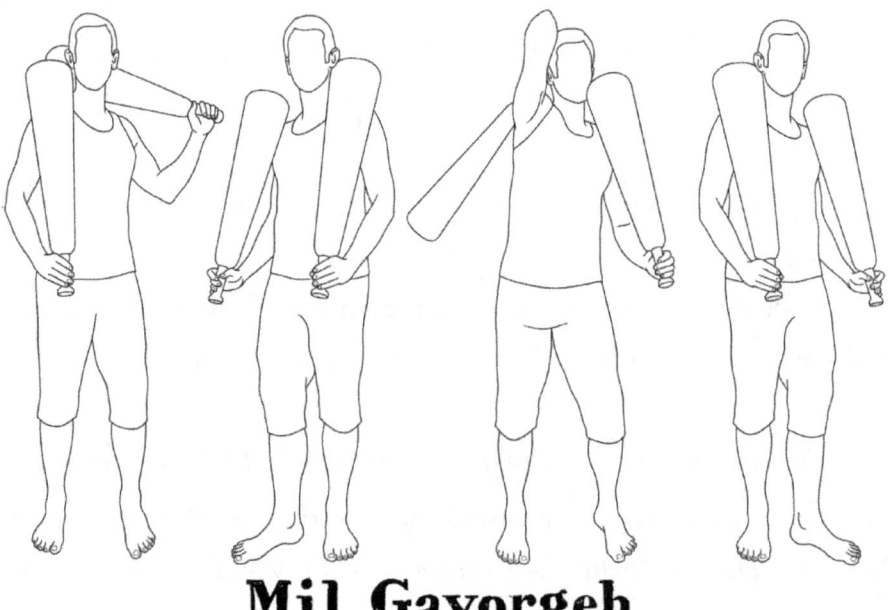

Mil Gavorgeh

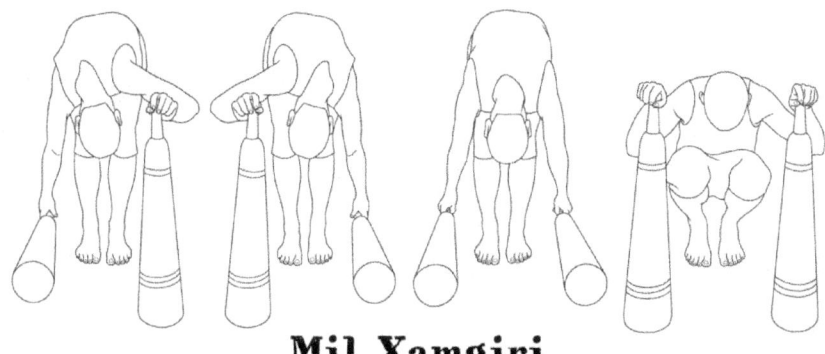

Mil Xamgiri

The body raises and the movement is repeated with the left *mil*. Then it is repeated with both mil. Finally, the *mil* are kept standing upright while a squat is performed, keeping the hands on the pommels of the *mil* at all times. This is done for several repetitions.

"He girded himself with God's glory and lifted his heavy mace to his shoulders, ready for battle." Šahnāme

After the *mil xamgiri*, the *šallāghi* ("whipping"), or *čakoši* ("hammer"), swings are performed. These are two-count swings with a similar technique to the *gavorgeh*. No footwork is performed, and the feet remain planted in the narrow position.

The *mil* are swung more rapidly with one going over the shoulder as soon as the other is returning to the front position. Unlike with the other exercises where they flow into each other, there is a marked break between the four-count and two-count.

The *mil* are always put down between the two types of swing, normally with the *mil xamgiri* between the two phases. The entire *milgiri* phase lasts about ten minutes.

After this, some *zurxāne* may allow *milbāzi* ("*mil* playing"). *Milbāzi* involves juggling two or more *mil*, and is usually performed with very light *mil* (two to six lbs) by younger members of the *zurxāne*. Some of the stronger, older members may use two normal sized *mil* and perform some basic throws also.

The complex throws and turns can be done with three to six *mil* (using one or both hands) and are extremely impressive. While there has been an attempt to contextualise this practice in the knightly tradition of the past, there is no evidence to support this claim. It is a likely a modern addition no earlier than the 20th century.

Milbāzi is a true piece of showmanship. It requires balance, poise, coordination and concentration. It is always done as a solo exercise in the centre of the *go'd* while the other athletes watch.

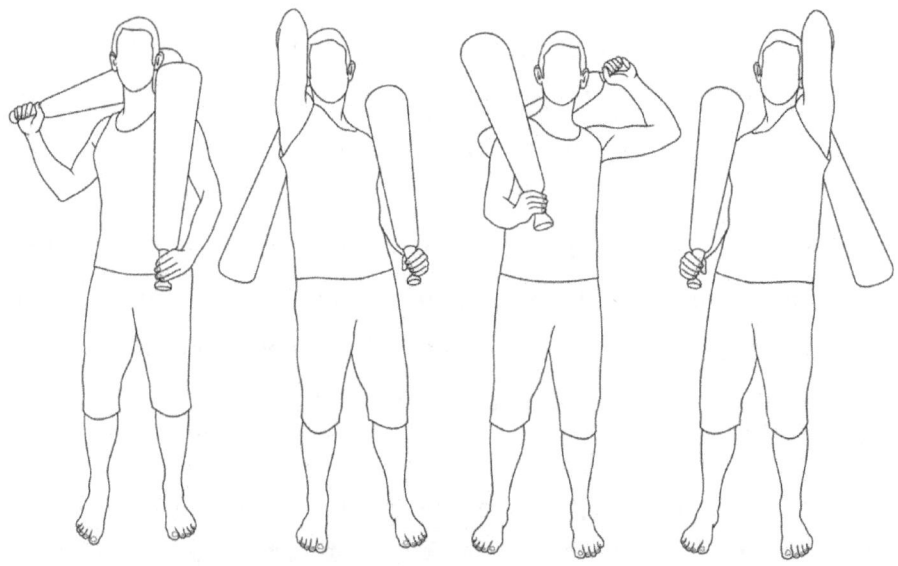

Mil Šallāghi

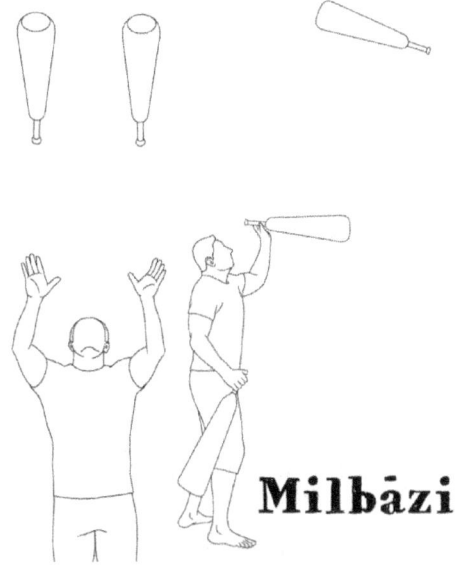

"For they are the bravest of the creation of both Spirits, the good, the strong, beneficent Fravašis of the Righteous." Fravardīn Yašt 13.76

There are countless complex variations of *milbāzi* moves. Throws are called *češme* and body turns are called *pič*. Two handed throws are *jofti* ("together") and different simultaneous throws with both hands are called *talfighi* ("combined").

The intricacies of *milbāzi* are complex and could fill a number of pages of a volume dedicated to the art. The majority of *zurxāne* in Iran do not have proficient *milbāzi* athletes, as the practice was frowned upon for a number of years by the governing body who proactively discouraged it. It is not particularly common to see *milbāzi* performed during the *varzeš-e pahlavāni* ritual in most *zurxāne*.

After the *mil* practice is over, the *mil* are returned to their positions on the edge of the *go'd* in order of seniority.

"Know that this is a war against Ahriman; keep yourselves ready, and live in the knowledge of God's protection. Whoever is killed in this battle will be received into paradise." Šahnāme

Pā Zadan

"The benefit of stepping and jumping on the stone ground is that it hardens the body whereas stepping and jumping on the wooden ground makes the body soft." Scroll of Puryā-ye Vali

After the mil have been replaced and the athletes have returned to their positions, the *pā zadan* ("footwork") begins. The *pā zadan* is aerobic conditioning for nimbleness, speed, and dexterity. The *miyāndār* once again asks permission and retakes his place in the centre of the *go'd*.

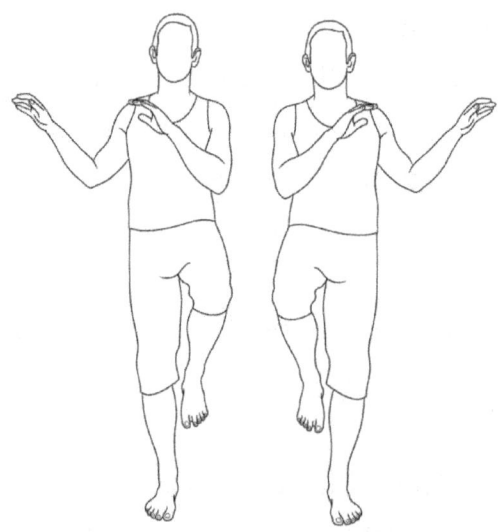

Pāy-e Dar Ja

First, the athletes begin a marching step called *pāy-e dar ja* ("stable steps"). The right heel is lifted, bending at the knee, while both arms sweep past the knees to the right. The hands swing to the left while the left heel is lifted. This is done in a steady and relaxed manner to a two-count rhythm.

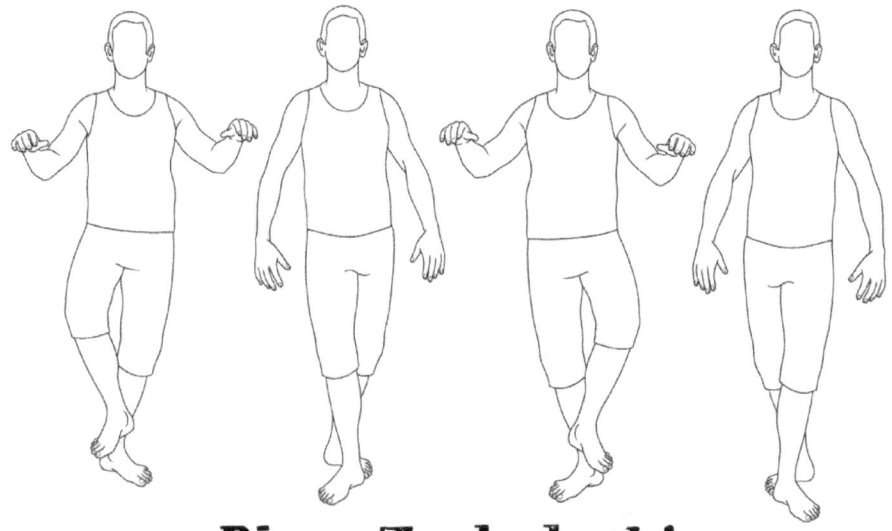

Pāy-e Zarbedaghi

Next the footwork transitions to *pāy-e zarbedaghi* ("cross-wise steps"). Both arms are raised upwards as each step rises and downwards as each step descends. The right leg lifts up with the knee bent and the foot pointing towards the ground. It is placed in front and slightly to the left of the left foot.

The left foot is then raised and put down in front and slightly to the right of the right foot. This is repeated for six to eight steps forward and then reversed to move backwards for the same number of steps, returning the athlete to his starting position. This forwards and then backwards movement is repeated a few times.

"The righteous souls pass over on the Chinwad bridge by spiritual flight and the power of good works; and they step forth up to the star, or to the moon, or to the sun station, or to the endless light. The soul of the wicked, owing to its falling

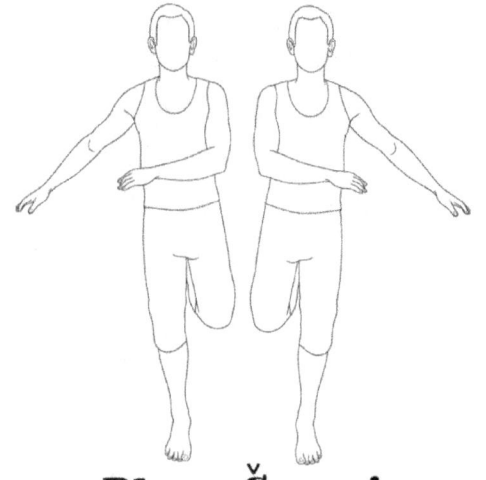

Pāy-e Šateri

from the bridge, its lying demon, and the pollution collected by its sin, they shall lead therefrom to the descent into the earth, as both ways lead from that bridge on the Daitih peak."
Dādēstān ī Dēnīg 34.3-4

The third set of steps is the *pāy-e šāteri* ("camel steps"). The *pāy-e šāteri* is used to slowly march around the *go'd* upon entry and again at the end of the *narmeš*, except vigorously. This third time it is used, it is performed with vigour to a two-count.

This then transitions into a four-count where the first three steps are the same marching feet as in the standard *šāteri*. On the four, both feet are jumped forward at the same time in a move called the *miyānkub zadan* ("knocking"). This is repeated a few times before it shifts to two *miyānkub* after three marching steps.

Finally, the *šāteri* ends with three *miyānkub* after three marching steps.

Next, the *miyānkub* are performed three times on the spot without the marching steps. This is done three times for a total of nine *miyānkub*. This phase of *miyānkub* is sometimes called *pāy-e jofti* ("feet together steps").

Following these *miyānkub*, the *pāy-e tabrizi* ("Tabrizi steps") are performed. These are straight leg kicking steps. The hands are held at chest height and then thrown down to the sides at the same time that the right leg is kicked up to waist height. The leg is fully extended 45 degrees to the right. This is repeated on the left and continued back and forth between legs to a two count.

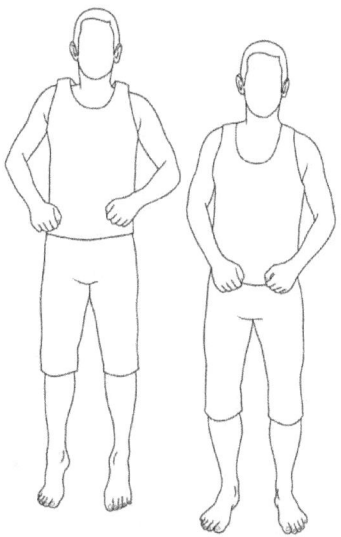

Miyānkub

"The Stranger, called by the name of Spirit, journeyed until he reached the country of Yūḥ (the Heaven of the Sun, the 4th Sphere). When he reached that heaven, he knocked on the door of that forbidden threshold."
'Abd al-Karīm al-Jīlī, **Universal Man**

Following on from the consecutive *tabrizi* is the single *tabrizi*. A single *tabrizi* step is performed on the right, followed by three light steps in the middle, making a four count. A single *tabrizi* is then kicked out to the left, followed by three steps in the middle.

This is done for several repetitions before transitioning to a double *tabrizi* where the right, then left is kicked out before three steps in the middle. Finally, a triple *tabrizi* is performed with the right, then the left; then the right is kicked before the three steps in the middle.

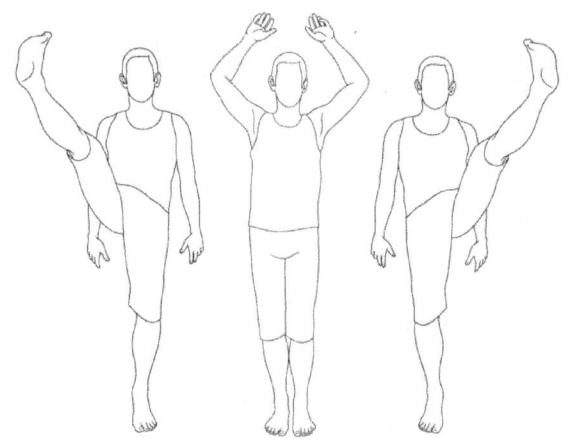

Pāy-e Tabrizi

Following straight on from the *tabrizi* is *pāy-e yā fattāḥ*. The phrase *yā fattāḥ* means "O opener" and is a call to God in his attribute as "opener of the gates." This step is sometimes referred to as *pāy-e yā Allāh*.

Three *tabrizi* are performed, followed by a set of three *miyānkub*. This then transitions into three *tabrizi* and two sets of *miyānkub*, before finally three *tabrizi* and three sets of *miyānkub*. This ends the main phase of the *pā zadan*, which lasts between five and ten minutes.

Another set of steps that is sometimes included in the *pā zadan* is the *pāy-e kermānšāhi* ("Kermānšāh steps"), where the right leg is kicked across to the left and the left leg is kicked to the right. While common in *zurxāne*, the *kermānšāhi* is not part of the official IZSF competition steps.

"Man alone can step out of the cosmos, and this possibility proves – and presupposes – that in a certain way he incarnates the Absolute." Frithjof Schuon, Stations of Wisdom

Čarx

"He should start to whirl around which has four effects on the body provided he starts to whirl around slowly and then whirl around fast... When he whirls around fast, he will become strong." Tumār-e Puryā-ye Vali

After the main segment of *pā zadan* is completed, the athletes begin the *čarx* ("whirling"). This spinning is traditionally said to help the blood circulate and strengthen the body above the waist, which is considered weaker than the lower body. It is said to be done for blood flow and brain health also.

The *čarx* originates on the battlefield. According to folkloric history, as a last resort when a soldier was outnumbered and surrounded on the battlefield, he would take up two swords and spin around to kill as many enemies as he could.

The *čarx* is performed by the junior members first, with the senior members going last. It begins with a *rajas xani* ("champion's boast"). Near the centre of the *go'd*, the *pahlavān* takes three steps while swinging his arms back and forth, then turns 60 degrees to the left and performed another three steps.

He turns left 60 degrees again followed by another three steps, thus creating an equilateral triangle around the centre of the *go'd*. He takes three steps back to the centre of the *go'd*, then three steps forward, before going through the process of stepping out an equilateral triangle again.

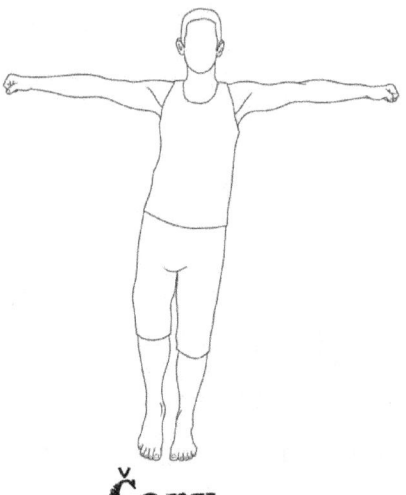

Čarx

"You are the kernel of the world in the midst thereof, know yourself that you are the world's soul." Mahmūd Šabestarī, Rose Garden of Secrets

After this, the athlete takes up the centre of the *go'd* to begin his *čarx*. While there are several variations and styles mixing jumps with the turns, the *čarx* at its core involves slow turns and fast turns. The aim is to remain spinning as close to the centre of the *go'd* as possible.

First, the *čarx-e čamani* ("grass-type whirling") is performed. The name implies the idea of going for a stroll and the *čamani* is a slow spin. The left foot is used as a supporting column, while the right foot pushes off the floor to turn the body in a anticlockwise direction.

The arms are held out to the sides at a 90-degree angle to the torso with the hands in loose fists. The head is held upright, and the face remains looking straight ahead, not moving with the turning of the body. The rotation is done at a slow and steady pace.

As the athlete builds up speed, he begins to enter the *čarx-e tiz* ("sharp whirling") phase. The athlete spins faster as the drum of the *moršed* speeds up. His aim should be to have maximum speed of rotation with minimal lift off the ground.

The supporting leg turns quickly also to help increase the speed. It is concluded by a full spin with both feet off the ground known as a *čarx-e takfar* ("single jump whirling").

"The warrior evokes in himself the transcendent power of destruction; he takes it on, becomes transfigured in it and free, thus breaking loose from all human bonds." Julius Evola, Metaphysics of War

After the most senior athlete who wishes to perform the *čarx* has completed his rotations, the final phase of the group training begins. The *pāy-e axār* ("last steps") are composed of two phases.

The first is *pāy-e owj* ("peak steps"). The move starts with a light hopping jump where the left leg remains straight and pointing at the floor, while the right knee comes up. Three steps are then taken forward, leading with the left leg, and the jump is repeated. Three steps, starting with the left, are taken backwards and the process is continued.

The next phase of the *owj* is two jumps before the steps. The hopping jump is performed like the first time, then the left leg comes up as if marching, before performing the same jump again. Then three steps are taken forward and the double jump repeated.

The final stage employs three hopping jumps on either end of the three steps forward and back.

The second *axār*, and final part of the entire group practice is *pāy-e tiz* ("sharp steps"). This involves jogging on the spot and kicking the heels back. The first part is three jogging steps with a slight pause before doing another three. Then four jogging steps are performed with a pause after the third and the fourth.

Next, five jogging steps are performed with a pause after the third, fourth and fifth. Finally, the jogging steps are performed continually until the *moršed* stops playing.

"The composition of man is the noblest of all, for one finds in him traces of the corporeal world as well as of the spiritual one, and it is in man that the arrangement of the powers is the most perfect. In other words, man combines the traces of the two universes and of the two worlds. Everything that is scattered in the world is reunited in him." Muḥammad al-Šahrastānī, The Book of Sects and Creeds

After the *čarx*, the *moršed* and *miyāndār* lead a prayer for the health and wellbeing of the *pahlavānān*, the audience, their families, the community at large, and the whole world. The prayer opens with the line "first and last of men in the world may you have a good and blessed ending." This does not only refer to a "good death," but to a healthy, long, and powerful life leading up to it.

The athletes then exit the *go'd* in order of seniority as the *moršed* beats a rhythm on the *zarb*. The *pahlavān* bends down, touching the *go'd* with his fingers, kisses them, and then touches his forehead as he did upon entering. He steps out with his left foot first, indicating his return to the profane world.

"And it is Light upon Light." Qoran 24.35

Kabbāde

"One should pull the kabbāde one hundred times." Tumār-e Puryā-ye Vali

Two iconic exercises of *varzeš-e pahlavāni* do not form part of the main practice, as they are individual arts. The use of the *kabbāde* (steel bow) and *sang* (wooden shields) are normally practiced either before the main group exercise, or after.

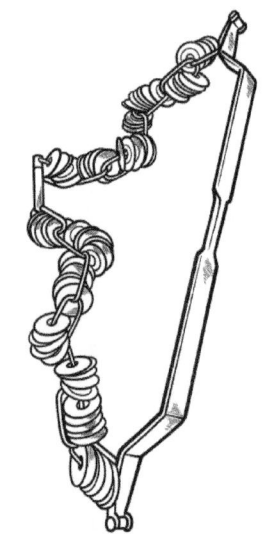

Serious *pahlavānān* will often exercise before the main practice, going for a run and doing warmups prior to their *kabbāde* or *sang* work. If performed during the main practice of *varzeš-e pahlavāni*, the most junior goes first, ending with the most senior. In this case the *xādem* ("servant") covers the athletes who are waiting to use the *kabbāde* with a towel so they don't get cold.

Kabbāde zadan (bow practice) is one of the least intuitive exercises in the *zurxāne*. The *kabbāde* is a steel or iron bow with a chain instead of a string. The chain also has metal coins on it to make a balanced weight between the bow and the string, as well as to help make the *kabbāde* "sing."

The *kabbāde* normally weighs between 26 and 48 lbs and is around 60 inches long. The *qabze* (handle) of the *kabbāde* is around 8 inches long. Originally, the *kabbāde* was a supple bow made of wood, but over time, the steel *kabbāde*, which retained the shape of a war bow, became the standard. There are two shapes of *kabbāde*: *kabbāde-ye moqavvas* (curved bow) and *kabbāde-ye čahrqoʾs* (with four curves). The latter is the more common.

"Summoning his last strength, he drew back the bowstring and released the arrow." *Šahnāme*

The *kabbāde* has an important place in the cultural milieu of Iran, as the bow and archery have a prominent place in Iranian history and mythology. Alongside the mace, the bow was the symbol of the Iranian noble warrior. In a famous section of the *Šahnāme* Rostam fires an arrow through a tree to kill Šaghad and avenge his own impending death.

In Iranian folklore, the boundary between Iran and their neighbouring enemy Tūrān was set by an arrow fired by Āraš-e Kamāngīr. The arrow fired by Āraš travelled for days before landing on the other side of the Oxus River in Afghanistan. Āraš has his roots in the *Avesta* where he is called Ərəxša and associated with Tištrya (the star Sirius) who is "as strong as an arrow."

Āraš is also the ancestral prototype for the ruling Aršak dynasty of the Parthian empire. The Parthians were skilled bowmen, inventing the tactic of feigning retreat on their horses, before turning their body backwards and firing at the advancing enemy: the eponymous "Parthian shot."

Athletes often kiss the handle of the *kabbāde* when they pick it up; then, holding the handle in the right hand with the *kabbāde* on the right-hand side of the body, the left hand is placed under the front of the bow. With a step forward, the *kabbāde* is swung forward and up above the head; the left hand then catches the second handle in the centre of the chain. The feet are brought close together in a narrow stance while the arms and body form a Y shape. This is the starting position for the *kabbāde zadan*.

"We sacrifice unto Tištrya, the bright and glorious star; who flies, towards the sea Vourukaša, as swiftly as the arrow darted through the heavenly space, which Ǝrəxša, the swift archer, the Arya amongst the Aryas whose arrow was the swiftest, shot from Mount Xšaotha to Mount Hvanvant." Tištar Yašt 8.6

The standard exercise with the *kabbāde* is the *yektaraf* ("one-sided") sway. The right heel is lifted slightly from the ground as the body is swayed slightly to the left. The right knee gently bends with this movement, but the hip does not move forward, remaining in line with the torso. At the same time, the right arm is extended as the left hand is held just above the head.

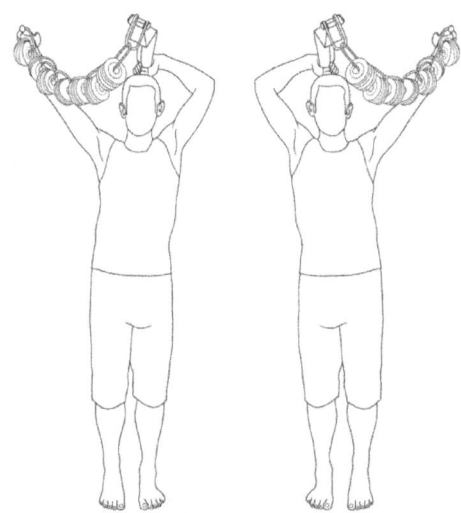

Kabbāde Yektaraf

The body then sways the other way as the right heel drops and the left heel lifts, and the arms shift position so that the right hand is above the head and the left is extended. Experienced athletes will also step forwards and backwards while doing this.

The movements are done rhythmically to the singing and playing of the *moršed*. If performed correctly, the *kabbāde* will "sing." It should make a jingling sound to the rhythm of the *moršed*. The rhythm of universal order can be discovered through the rhythm of the *kabbāde*.

"He created a secret artifice and commissioned a wizard to make an iron bow weighing more than fifty mann. On the iron, he had attached wood and horn. The ends of the handle were decorated with ivory. From a chain he made a string for the bow." Garšāspnāme

The more experienced athletes may be able to perform the *dotarafe* ("two-sided") sway. This is the same as the *yektaraf*, except the hand of the bent arm crosses the head to the shoulder of the extended arm. This is a more difficult manoeuvre, requiring great shoulder and upper arm strength, so it is not encouraged among beginners.

Another experienced move is the *ru beruye sine* ("facing chest"), in which the *kabbāde* is held in front of the chest and pulled open with both arms like a chest expander. This is a difficult exercise and fairly uncommon.

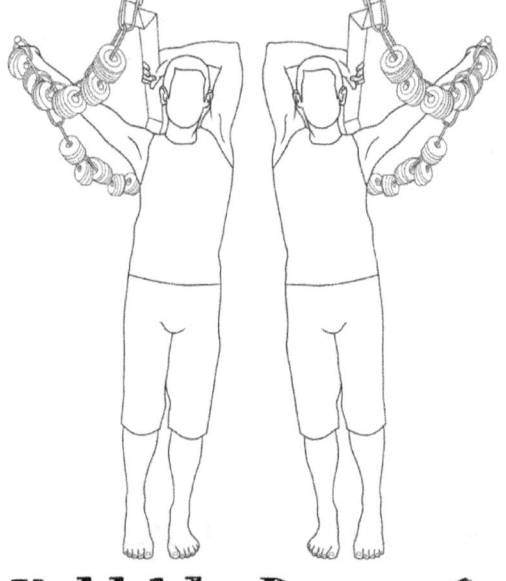

The *čarx-e kabbāde* ("whirling with kabbāde")

Kabbāde Dotarafe

is done with the *kabbāde* placed across the shoulders before performing the *čarx*. This is often part of the fancy *širin kari* ("sweet work") moves used during *kabbāde* competition.

Much like with the *mil*, the *kabbāde* specialist knows several showy moves that involve spinning the *kabbāde* and moving it around the body with skill and poise. The *kabbāde* builds strength and endurance in the shoulders, arms, back, chest and grip.

"I concentrated my attention on the constellation of the Bear and I observed that it formed seven apertures through which God was showing himself to me." Rūzbihān Baqlī, **Unveiling of Secrets**

Sang

"They say that Pahlavān Širdel had two sang made of marble... He took them and trained with them fifty times each morning and fifty times each evening." Tumār-e Puryā-ye Vali

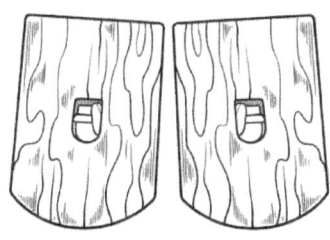

The *sang* are wooden shields, which are pressed upwards while lying prone on the ground. The word literally means "stones," as the original iteration were made of stone. The original name was *sang-e zur* ("stones of power"), but in their current form they are a representation of the *separ* ("shield"). Considered the "first tool" of *varzeš-e pahlavāni*, the sang are usually around 44 inches tall, 32 inches wide, and a minimum of 2.5 inches thick. The weight is added by increasing the thickness rather than the other aspects.

A pair usually weighs between 66 lbs (33 lb each) and 220 lbs. The purpose of the *sang* is to build excellent pushing and pressing strength, while in a state of motion, rather than in a static position.

The sang are shaped like flat shields with a curved bottom edge and a flat top. The handle is perfectly central to the weight distribution, making a completely balanced tool. There is often a felt disc on the thumb side of the handle to prevent chaffing.

"In taking the sang, the beginner should lie on his back on the ground. The place on the ground should be hard, not soft. Because if it is hard, it hardens the body." Tumār-e Puryā-ye Vali

As the *moršed* performs a song called the *gol-e sang,* the athlete prostrates in front of the *sang,* kissing the ground to show humility and gratitude to God. The athlete then turns his body to the right to lie in a prone position facing the sky to begin *sang giri* ("sang practice"). Sometimes he lies on a carpet or *long.*

The arms are then extended back to grasp the handles of the *sang,* which are normally propped up at the edge of the *go'd*. The *sang* are then lifted up into a top press position above the chest. The arms are extended with the *sang* lining up along the arms on each side.

The two flat edges of the *sang* should be about an inch apart. The spine and head should touch the ground with both shoulders raised up. The feet are placed together with the right big toe crossing over the left big toe.

This is the starting position of the *sanggereftan-e jofti* ("paired taking of *sang*") or *sanggiri-ye jofti* ("paired *sang* workout") – the double press. From here, the *sang* are lowered, allowing them to go

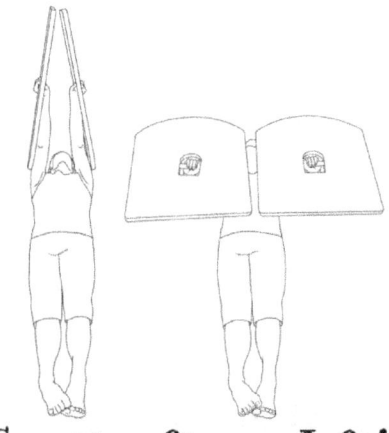

Sanggereftan-e Jofti

into a horizontal position as the elbows touch the ground 90 degrees from the torso, forming a T position with the body. The head raises at this bottom position, looking through the space between the *sang*.

The *sang* should not touch the body. The sang are then pressed up into the top position with the head lowering to the ground. This is performed seventeen times.

> *"Praying to god for strength, he set his hands to the stone and lifted it."* Šahnāme

After completing the seventeen presses of the *sanggereftan-e jofti* the second phase of the *sang giri* begins. The *sanggereftan-e qaltān* ("turning *sang* lifts") start with the knees touching and the legs raised upwards. The knees are bent with the shins in a horizontal position.

As one sang remains at the top position, the other sang is lowered into the bottom position as the body turns in that direction. At this bottom position, the legs straighten to the side to put the body in an L position.

The legs are then bent again. The knees remain in contact as they arch to the other side, pressing the lowered *sang* upright. The upright *sang* is lowered on the other side.

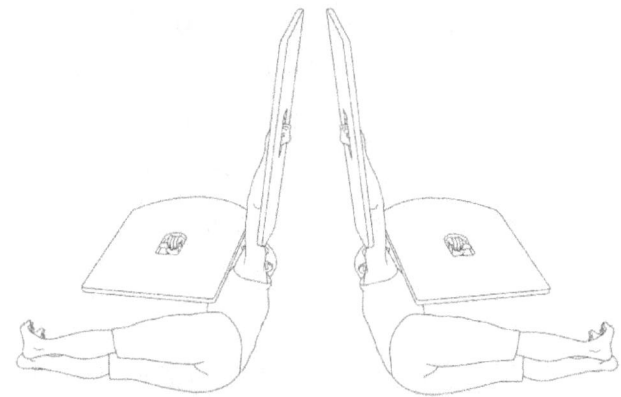

Sanggereftan-e Qaltān

This movement is repeated continually until the athlete is no longer able to continue. In competition, the number of turning repetitions is what counts as the competitor's score. One repetition is a turn to the right and to the left.

The skilled *sang* specialist also has an arsenal of *širin kari* moves that involve turning the *sang* at different angles on the bottom and top positions to show his flair in competition. The *sang* may also be used while standing to perform a shoulder press variation.

Some say that the sang have a link to the pilgrimage to Mecca. When Muslims go on their pilgrimage, they throw stones against the devil after having returned from walking seven times around the Ka'ba. The stones are cast against a person's own ego, also considered to be the devil that lives within us. Therefore, the *sang* can represent the casting of stones against the ego.

"We worship Ahura-created Vərəthragna who makes men virile, who makes men strong." Wahrām Yašt 14.28

Košti-ye Pahlavāni

"Praise to God Almighty that we do not wrestle for money and do not wrestle for the prizes, nor do we wrestle for the titles. We wrestle for the glory of Iran and her people."
Pahlāvan Bozorg Razzāz

Košti-ye pahlavāni ("champion wrestling") is the culminating activity that all other exercises lead to. Most *zurxāne* no longer practice *košti* at the end of the exercises, but it once was part of every practice. Each of the moves were geared towards wrestling, from the sprawling *šeno* and positional *narmeš*, to the hand-fighting and grip working of the *mil*; and from the footwork of the *pā zadan* and *čarx* to, the arm strength of the *kabbāde* and *sang*. The separation of the two exercises in most *zurxāne* has led to a disconnect in culture and a decline in both aspects of the *zurxāne* practice (*varzeš-e pahlavāni* and *košti-ye pahlavāni*).

Wrestling, which is deeply embedded in the Iranian psyche, was particularly part of Parthian culture and was associated with feasting and celebration. This was inherited by the Sasanian dynasty, and is reflected in the artefacts found in Northeastern Iran of Sassanian origin that depict wrestling, in particular two 7th century silver bowls that depict wrestlers.

One is in the Sacker Museum in Washington DC and the other in the Cleveland Museum of Art. The term *pahlavān* is testament to this, as it derives from the word "Parthian." Over the course of time, the word came to mean "wrestler."

"I never try my strength with wrestlers or drink with my friends till I can drink no more." Fakhr al-Din Gorgāni, Vis va Rāmin

Košti-ye pahlavāni is a form of belt wrestling where the *tombān* (wrestling pants) are worn. The wrestlers can catch any hold they like on the upper body and may grip the belt and pants also. The aim is to throw the opponent so that any part of his back touches the ground.

The term *košti*, which denotes wrestling, derives from the Middle Persian word *kust* ("side"). *Košti* is the name also given to the sacred thread worn around the waist by Zoroastrians. According to the 17th century dictionary *Borhān-e Qāte'*, one of the meanings of *košti* is "*a rope that the wrestlers of Xorāsān tie around their waists.*"

Belt wrestling is not specific to the Iranians. It is found throughout the Indo-European diaspora as well as beyond into East Asia. Reflections are found in Icelandic *glíma*, Swiss *schwingen*, Japanese *sumo*, and Korean *ssireum*.

The ancient Greeks also practiced belt wrestling prior to transtitioning to the fully naked *pálē* variant.

The Greek historian Thucydides states, *"Formerly, even in the Olympic contests, the athletes who contended wore belts across their middles; and it is but a few years since that the practice ceased. To this day among some of the barbarians, especially in Asia, when prizes for boxing and wrestling are offered, belts are worn by the combatants."* (The History of the Peloponnesian War, I.6.4-6).

"Iranian men tussle with each other to the end of their lives." Terence O'Donnell, Garden of the Brave in War

The Iranian epic tradition is punctuated with wrestling, once again tying the tradition to the Parthian/Saka culture of the Xorāsāni Sistān region, or *Airyanəm Vaējah* ("expanse of the Aryans"). In the *Šahnāme*, the belt used in wrestling is called *dovāl* or *kamar*, and many battles are settled in the work through wrestling.

Rostam wrestles both his son Sohrāb and Pulādvand. In both instances, they seize each other by the belt. Bizhan seizes Humān's neck with his left hand, his thigh with his right hand, lifts him up, throws him down, and then severs his head with his dagger. Kay Khosrow seizes Šideh's neck with his left hand and his back with his right hand, lifts him up, and flings him to the ground so hard that all his vertebrae are shattered and his leg is broken. Dārāb, the son of Queen Homāy, is an unbeatable wrestler.

In the final wrestling scene of the *Šahnāme*, the ruler of Iran, Bahrām Gur travels to the court of an Indian king. After drinking, he challenges one of the court wrestlers to a bout and wears a garment called an *ezār* which is described much like a *langot* (loin cloth) which is still worn by Indian wrestlers today. The fight is reminiscent of the ancient Indian style of *mallayuddha* and ends with Bahrām breaking the wrestler's bones.

The wrestling motif of heroes is continued in later Iranian epics such as the *Garshāspnāme, Kok Kuhzādnāme, Borzunāme, Šahryārnāme, Bahmannāme, Sāmname, Xāvarānnāme, and Rostamnāme*. A wrestling scene is found in almost every Iranian epic.

"[Khosrow] seized his opponent's neck with his left hand, his thigh with his right, and lifted him up and found him against the ground." Šahnāme

In South Asia, the name 'Rustam' signifies the epitome of physical strength, with the title *Rustam-i Hind* ("Rostam of India") used for the national wrestling champion up until Indian independence in 1947. It was in the 1940s that *košti-ye pahlavāni* began to disappear from the *zurxāne* with the introduction of international freestyle and Greco-Roman wrestling to Iran. The loss of the link between the *zurxāne* and *košti* has contributed to the decline of both institutions.

Traditionally, at the end of the *varzeš-e pahlavāni* practice, the *miyāndār* would ask the *pahlavānān* "what should we do now?" To which the answer was "*koštigiri*" ("wrestling") or *košti gereftan* ("to take wrestling"). The best *koštigir* ("wrestler") would then take the centre of the *go'd* and await challenges. As the wrestling was done, the others would watch.

After a successful win, the two wrestlers in the centre would shake hands and kiss each other on the cheek to denote no hard feelings were held. During the bouts, the *moršed* would chant the *golrizān* ("pouring flowers" or "flower of wrestling"). Upon completion of the wrestling, the athletes would leave the *go'd*.

"The master, lifting him up with his hands from the ground, raised him above his head and then threw him down." Sa'dī Shīrāzī, Golestān 1.27

While *košti-ye pahlavāni* has declined, it still forms part of the national *varzeš-e pahlavāni* competitions. The various regional variations, such as the *bāchukheh* jacket wrestling of the Xorāsān region, still survive in local tournaments. Wrestling is considered the national sport of Iran and when moves were made to eliminate it from the Olympics, the Iranians were the loudest voice against its removal.

"I trample on all unjust desires and renounce whatever is from Ahriman and not from God." Šahnāme

Competition

"Now we shall see to whom the Lord of the sun and the moon will give victory." Šahnāme

Aside from traditional wrestling competitions across Iran, there are *varzeš-e pahlavāni* competitions that are comprised of both group and individual categories. The competitions occur throughout the year and often coincide with significant days of the Islamic religious calendar. Individual categories are: heavy *mil* swings based on number of repetitions, *milbāzi* based on skill and variations, *sang* based on repetitions and variations, *kabbāde* based on repetitions and variations, *čarx* based on time and form, and *košti-ye pahlavāni*.

The team categories are based on synchronisation between team members, synchronisation between team and *moršed*, synchronisation between *miyāndār* and *moršed*, form and execution of basic technique, and variation and innovation of movement. These competitions fall under the auspices of the International Zurkhaneh Sports Federation. In recent years, the IZSF has worked to bring awareness of *varzeš-e pahlavāni* to the world, leading to foreign teams participating in Iranian competitions. This has had some limited success, with the sport remaining relatively obscure outside of the immediate area of Iran.

"This is the soul of al-insan al-kamil, the Perfect Man, as man is meant to be, the microcosm of the whole universe, who contains all that is in the universe." Šehāb-al-dīn Yaḥyā Sohravardī, The Shape of Light

Regimen

"The good, strong, beneficent Fravašis of the Righteous I praise... who bring much, who come powerfully, who come themselves, who come swiftly, who come strongly, who come at the call, who are to be invoked at bloody fights, who are to be invoked at battles..." Fravardīn Yašt 13.21-23

In the absence of a dedicated *zurxāne,* the WarYogin must build an inner House of Strength alone or with his dedicated *männerbund*. He must create his own routines that incorporate the exercises of *varzeš-e pahlavāni,* which are most pertinent to him with the tools available.

He must be creative with his resources and craft that which he cannot obtain, and substitute appropriately. A *taxte-ye šeno* can be easily constructed with little to no woodworking skills. The *sang* and *kabbāde* exercises can be emulated with dumbbells if required. Heavy clubs or even larger hammers can take the place of *mil* if necessary. While the original tools are ideal, the WarYogin never allows perfect to be the enemy of good.

If one were to break down the full practice into digestible parts that could compliment other modalities of training over a weekly schedule, the *šeno* exercises would form the first day, with all four variations making a "push-up day." This could be supplemented with *mil* work, but if making a more concise daily program, then it may be best to split the two.

"Each of us carries in himself the Image of his own world, his imago mundi, and projects it into a more or less coherent universe, which becomes the stage on which his destiny is played out." Henry Corbin, Avicenna and the Visionary Recital

The next day, following the *šeno* day, may focus solely on the *narmeš* stretches, much as they follow the *šeno* work in the *zurxāne*. This active rest day would allow for muscle recovery as well as work on range of motion and joint health. Without this practice, the heavier work of the *sang*, heavy *mil*, and *kabbāde* can be a strain on the body. The *pā zadan* footwork could be added to the *narmeš* if one were seeking to combine recovery and aerobic work.

The next day in the routine would be a *mil* day if not combined with the *šeno*. This would ensure that plenty of time was allotted to technical *mil* work. First several sets of four-count *gavorgeh*, enable focus on technique and assessment of movement. Then, two-count *šallāghi* can be performed to build rotational endurance and strength.

After this, the fancy *širin kari* swings can be experimented with for mental exercise. *Mil xamgiri* can be performed for some light squat work also.

"His shadow on earth is as that of Mount Qāf, his spirit is as a Simurgh soaring on high." Jalāl al-Dīn Muḥammad Rūmī, Masnavi 1.10

If the *pā zadan* has not been combined with the *narmeš*, then it can form the foundation of a "cardio day." This could include other aerobic and anaerobic exercises such as running, jumping rope, or other common modalities of exercise. *Pā zadan* could also be used to warmup before a primary sporting activity like grappling or striking.

The *sang* and *kabbāde* (or their equivalents) could be combined into an "arm and shoulder strength day." These are good tools to finish up a week of training on, as they can be used for a final "burn out." The *sang* in particular require a grind mentality, which enables the WarYogin to push beyond his self-imposed limitations.

Finally, as the traditional *varzeš-e pahlavāni* included wrestling, it is highly recommended that grappling and/or striking form a core part of the WarYogin's practice. These exercises are all designed to enhance combat sports. To use them in conjunction with martial arts is a powerful holistic practice.

"In the traditional world we encounter the interpretation of life as a perennial struggle between metaphysical powers, between Uranian forces of light and order, on the one hand, and telluric, dark forces of chaos and matter on the other. Traditional man yearned to fight this battle and to triumph in both the inner and outer worlds.

"A true and just war on the external plane reproduced in other terms the same struggle that had to be waged within: it was a struggle against forces and people that in the external world presented the same traits as the powers the single individual needed to subjugate and dominate internally, until a pax triumphalis was achieved." Julius Evola, Men Among the Ruins

Afterword

"Light the fire that will deliver us both from darkness." Šahnāme

The last flickers of the warrior traditions of the Indo-European people are struggling to remain alight. In this dark age of "mixture" we need heroes more than ever before in the history of humanity.

It is up to a new generation to take the flame that remains within them and feed it, growing it into a blazing torch that they can use to light an unquenchable inferno. Without you, this fire that has burned since the dawn of the Golden Age will be extinguished, leaving the world dark. An easy target for the forces of dissolution and decay.

"Cause the litany of Light to ascend. Cause the people of Light to triumph. Guide the Light towards the Light." Šehāb-al-dīn Yaḥyā Sohravardī

The battle between Light and Darkness has been fought for aeons. It has been fought since the creation of the Cosmos. The problem we face today is that one side has almost forgotten it is at war. The forces of Darkness never forget.

They work each day towards their goal of domination. To do this, they need simply for the Army of Light to forget. They need the flames within each of its warriors to die out. So long as one remains burning, the Darkness cannot win.

"When Ahriman is exterminated from the bodies of men he is destroyed from the whole of this world, and the good spirits will then predominate in human bodies." Dēnkard 6.265

In order to be a force of good in the world, each man must wage war against his lower Ahrimanic self. He must purge himself of the darkness within and strive ever upwards, reaching towards the light of the higher Self.

It is only through continual war against what is dark and chaotic that the WarYogin may rise. Through his struggle, others find their way and the warband of Mithra increases, becoming an unstoppable force fighting together to restore order and bring Light to the cosmos.

"Thereby follow days of strength, thus there will be days of victory!" Mihr Yašt 10.117

Appendix I

Excerpt from John Chardin, The Travels of Sir John Chardin in Persia, first published 1686

Wrestling is the Exercise of People in a lower Condition; and generally Speaking, only of People who are Indigent. They call the Place where they Show themselves to Wrestle, *Zour Kone,* that is to say, *The House of Force.* They have of'em in all the Houses of their great Lords, and especially those of the Governours of Provinces, to Exercise their People. Every Town has besides Companies of those Wrestlers for Show.

They call the Wrestlers Pehelvon, a Word which signifies Brave, Intrepid. They perform their exercises to divert People; for this is a Show, as I have said, and thus it is, They strip themselves Naked, only with their Shoes on, made of Leather, that fit them very exactly, oil'd and greas'd, and a Linnen Cloth about their Wast greas'd and oil'd likewise. This is, that the Adversary may have less to take hold of, because if he should touch there, his Hand would slip, and he would lose his Strength.

The two Wrestlers being Present upon an even Sand, a little Tabour, that always plays during the time of Wrestling, to animate them, gives the Signal. They begin by making a thousand Bravadoes and Rodomontades; then they promise each other fair Play, and shake Hands.

That being done, they strike at each others' Buttocks, Hips, and Thighs, keeping time with the little Tabour; then they shake Hands again, and strike at each other as before, three times together. This is as if it were for the Ladies, and to recover their Breath; after that, they close, making a great Out-cry, and strive with all their Might to overthrow their Man.

The Victory is never judg'd to signifie any thing, till the Man be laid flat upon his Belly, stretch'd all along the ground.

Appendix II

Excerpt from Carsten Niebuhr, Account of travels to Arabia and other surrounding lands, first published 1774

The Persians have public houses called Surchône (House of Strength) where anyone can go to publicly display their powers. When I first visited such a Surchône, I found the air there so impure that I thought it advisable to leave quickly. However, I ventured a second visit, and this time I stayed so long that I believe I can give my readers a clear idea of the physical exercises that are undertaken here.

The building was only small, but built high and strong. At each of the four sides was a niche or open chamber. The space in the middle was only for those who wished to show their skill or practice.

The door to this scene was small and low, and there was no window opening in the whole building; only at the top of the vault was a hole through which some light could fall; and as this was not sufficient, the scene had to be lighted with lamps. In short, it seemed that this building had only been designed to keep out all draughts.

This was of course necessary. But up in the vault one would have to make more draft holes and thereby clean the house of the bad fumes, which are not only a nuisance to those who are gathering here, but are also certainly harmful to their health.

I sat in a booth with a few spectators. The nobles and the merchants, who came here to practice, sat down in two other niches and first smoked a pipe of tobacco, like figure *a* on page 560, where I have tried to depict the whole spectacle. You could also get coffee here.

Three musicians sat in the fourth niche. One of them played a kind of zither, the second played a little drum, without which the Orientals never sing or dance, and the third sometimes sang a Persian song. When the aficionados had drunk their coffee and didn't want to smoke any more, one after the other, they undressed and jumped into the middle of the square, completely naked except for a pair of tight leather trousers that were fastened with a belt around the waist.

If someone was already very practiced in his art, he stood up on his hands with his feet in the air like figure *b*. Soon after, however, he stands on his feet and prays with his face turned towards Mecca. Because the Mohammedans are supposed to pray first in everything they do, and so they don't forget that duty when they start this kind of amusement. Most immediately said their prayers, throwing their faces to the ground as usual, figure *c*.

The first exercise undertaken is illustrated at *d* and *e*, in so far as such arts can be illustrated. The whole company stood side by side on their hands and knees. When one was still a beginner, he stood about like *d*, but a master stretched his hands and feet as far apart as possible, not touching the earth with his abdomen. Figure *e*. In this position, without moving their hands or feet, everyone had to draw a circle with their head, as it were, and if this was done twice, also depict the diameter.

The more often one can repeat this exercise, the greater his art. I certainly believe that some repeated it over 60 times. Everything happened to the music and very rhythmically. Then some took a large piece of round wood in each hand and threw it on the shoulder (*f*). All they had to do was move the wood from the front to the back on the shoulder according to the beat.

Afterwards, some jumped their feet against the board that they had placed at an angle against the wall, as in *g*. Others, who were already more practiced, put their feet higher as in *h*, and finally some, who had advanced even higher in their art, put their hands on the ground as in the figure *b*.

It was inevitable that people would sweat profusely after such exercises. So those who wanted to pay for it sat in a niche and let a servant rub them dutifully (*i*): he also worked to the beat and sometimes gave the person who had put himself under his hands a hard blow with his flat hand on the wet back. Afterwards he squeezed and stretched all his limbs.

Then everyone began to dance; not in the European manner, where one is taught to put the feet out, carry the body straight and light, but each hopped for himself, some round in a circle (*k*) and others against a wall (*l*), all soon on one foot, then on the other, and this as hard as possible to shake the body well. Some lay on their backs (*m*) with pillows under their heads and arms to lift two thick and heavy pieces of wood to the beat. Only a few were able to do this exercise because it requires extraordinary strength.

The Master sat and counted aloud the number of times the student lifted the pieces of wood; it is therefore easy to think that those who follow always strive to surpass those who have gone before. Thereupon all lined up and the Master made before them a speech or lengthy prayer, often naming Ali, Hassan and Hussein, with all wrestlers or fighters appearing to be very reverent.

It was not possible to draw and describe all the different body positions that I saw in the following exercises. I only got one displayed at *n* and it didn't last long. The feet always stayed in one place, but the body moved now up, now down, now forwards, now backwards.

Then some began to wrestle in pairs, and not without compliments beforehand. Among others, two clasped their hands together and crossed them in front of their foreheads like *o*, which I took as a greeting. Then they sat down on the ground facing each other.

Each sought how best to attack his opponent; and when they got into a hand-to-hand fight, they struggled around, now on their knees, now on their feet, until one was lying on the ground. Then the vanquished kissed the hand of the victor in a very respectful manner. Here there were no thrusts or blows, as when the English box each other. However, some felt their arms and legs when they left the square, as if their limbs needed rest. One of them gradually threw to the ground all those who wanted to test their strength against him; and when at last no one appeared, he demanded a small tip from the spectators.

If anyone can bring proof that he had made it known in a Mohammedan capital, for example in Isfahan, Constantinople or Delhi, that at a certain time he wished to wrestle with the strongest and that no one could be found who would have thrown him to the ground, he is at liberty to have a lion carved in stone placed on his grave. I have seen two such graves at Shiraz, one in a burial ground near the newly created garden of Karim Khan and the other near the Shah Cheragh Mosque. I suspected at first that those who were buried here must be great lords who had shown extraordinary bravery either in war or in the lion-hunt, but afterwards heard that their greatest bravery was in wrestling. Who knows how often great scholars who want to explain antiquities make equally great mistakes. In Sheikh Saadi's Persian Rose Garden there are some nice children's fables, which the European reader will now understand better.

At Shiraz there are three such public Surchône, where not only persons of the middle and lower rank, but sometimes also noble military and civil servants, gather to strengthen their bodies by such exercises. The great gentlemen sometimes have rooms in their houses set up for this purpose, in order to wrestle there with their friends and acquaintances. This physical exercise is practiced by the noble Persians in the morning; in the afternoon they are on horseback.

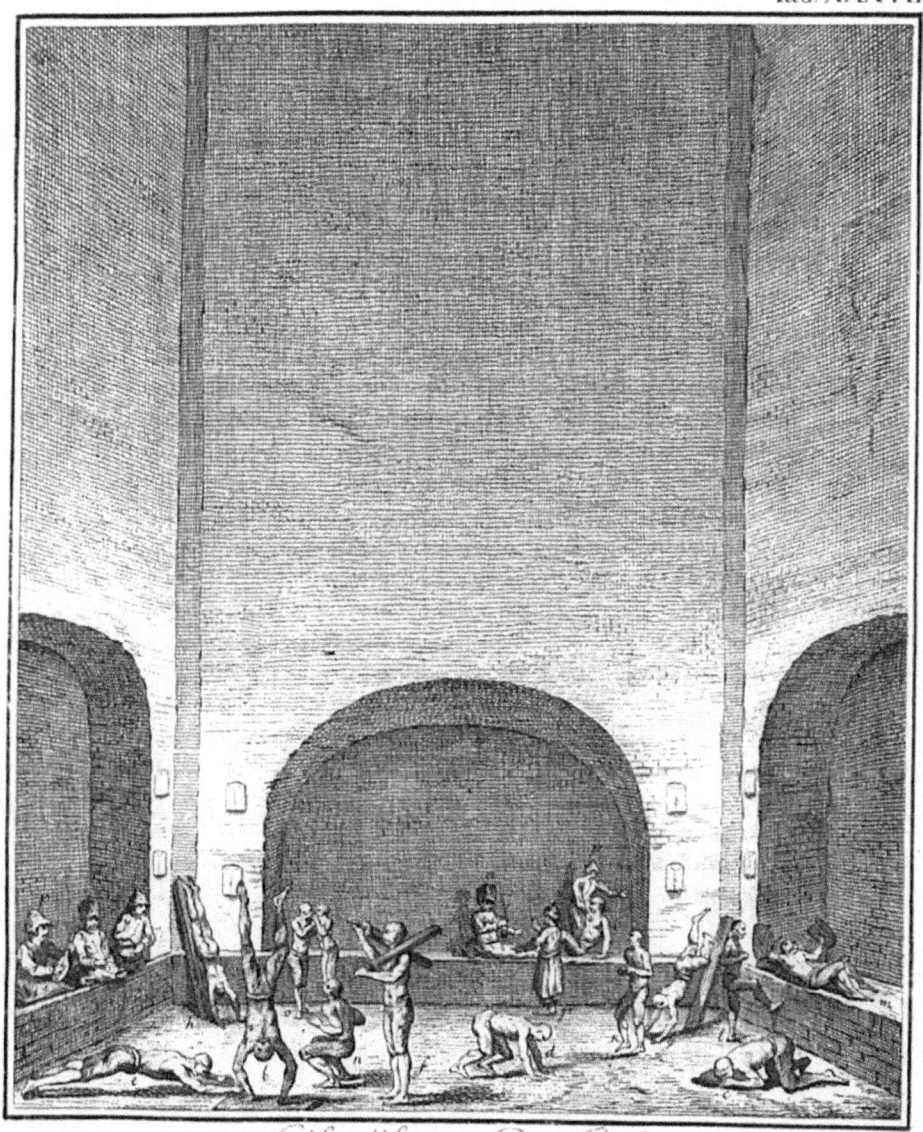

Tab. XXXVII.

Leibesübungen der Perser.

Glossary

Aēšma: The state of furor that warriors cultivated for battle – also called "fury."

Ahura Mazdā ("Wise Lord"): Originally an epithet which became the name of the god, this development from Vourunā (Vedic Varuṇa) – with some elements of the Sky Father Dyaoš (Vedic Dyáuṣ) – became the "one god" of Mazdāism and later Zoroastrianism (also as Ohrmazd). Mazdā's element is ātar ("fire") in Avestan lore; this diverges from Varuṇa whose element is water. Like Varuṇa however, Mazdā tends to Cosmic Order: Aša (Vedic Ṛta).

Ahuras ("Lords"): Older, priestly gods who used magical powers to intervene in the world and assumed the role of the good gods in pre-Islamic Iran.

Aŋgra Mainyu ("Hostile Spirit"): The great evil spirit of Mazdāism and later Zoroastrianism (also as Ahriman) who played the demonic adversary of Ahura Mazdā (Ohrmazd).

Arədvī Sūrā Anāhitā: Invoked more concisely as Anāhitā, this is the Celestial River goddess that feeds all rivers and the only deity to be worshipped in images.

Aryan: A designation not only common to the various Iranian people, but all Indo-Europeans (as evidenced in the Indian "ā́rya" and Greek "aristoi").

Aryāna Vaējah ("Cradle of the Aryans"): Where the Kayānids (legendary hero kings) were created, and the place of the liturgies of Ahura Mazdā. It is also where the first king Yima built the vara, and the elite shelter to repopulate the world after the Cosmic Winter.

Aša: "Truth," "Cosmic Order," and Right Action.

Asman ("Stone"): The stone vault of the heavens (the sky).

Avesta: Zoroastrianism's holy scripture.

Bundahišn: A late Zoroastrian creation text.

Čarx ("Whirling"): Spinning traditionally said to help the blood circulate and strengthen the body above the waist, which is considered weaker than the lower body. It is said to be done for blood flow and brain health also.

Činvatō Pərətu ("Requiter's Crossing"): The bridge of judgement souls must pass over to be ruled on by the god Mithra.

Daēvas ("Shining Ones"): Martial, upstart gods characterised by their strength and moral ambiguity. In Iran they eventually became evil, with the term also designating demons.

Druj: "Falsehood," "disorder," and the anticosmic principle.

Fravaši: Ancestor spirits unique to Iran, with some characteristics of the Vedic Pitṛ (ancestors), as well as embodying the Spirit of the manifold soul. Fighting alongside Mithra and his elite command, they are his warriors: his *männerbund*.

Gaokarena: "White Haoma."

Garōdəmāna ("House of Song") or Asar-Rōšnīh ("Realm of Light"): The Throne of Ahura Mazdā.

Gāthās: The oldest section of the Avesta.

Go'd ("Hollow" or "Deep"): A sacred space in which activities of the zurxāne take place. It is a sunken pit in the center of the room that is either hexagonal, octagonal, square, or round.

Haoma: The juice of a plant personified in a god called Haoma (Pahlavi: Hōm). The identity of haoma is unknown, but could have been the ephedra plant, which fits the description of the plant and effects of consuming it. Haoma was intoxicating but did not make one drunk, and was a stimulant taken before battle, enhancing mental capabilities and perception.

Harā Bərəzaitī: The Cosmic Mountain Range.

Jihad ("Holy War" and "Path of God"): Islamic concept – dependent on its inheritance from Iranian tradition – of a violent religious campaign. Can be divided into "greater" and "lesser" forms.

Kabbāde: A steel or iron bow with a chain instead of a string. The chain also has metal coins on it to make a balanced weight between the bow and the string, as well as to help make it "sing."

Košti-ye Pahlavāni ("Champion Wrestling"): A form of belt wrestling and the culminating activity that all other exercises lead to. Most zurxāne no longer practice this at the end of the exercises, but it once was part of every practice.

Mehr Yašt: A hymn to Mithra.

Mehragān: The the autumnal equinox festival of Mithra, symbolic of completion and the end of the current cycle. This celebration is ancient and deeply embedded in the Indo-Iranian religion, and the only one where Ahura Mazdā is not invoked as part of the ceremony.

Mil: Wooden clubs.

Mithra: This Ahura is a strong warrior associated with fire, bull sacrifice, and contracts. Priginally a priestly deity, he transitioned from a god of the priestly caste to one of the warriors, taking over much of the role of the daēva Indara.

Mithrayazna ("Worship of Mithra"): The esoteric religion of the pre-Islamic Iranian Elite, with Mithra being referred to as bagā vazrakā ("great god").

Miyāndār: Drawn from the senior members of the zurxāne, this pahlavān leads the exercises from the centre of the go'd. He is responsible for keeping the pace within the go'd and communicating with the moršed on both a verbal and non-verbal level, as well as demonstrating correct technique to the novices.

Mojāhedīn: Holy warriors.

Moršed ("Master" or "Guide"): Responsible for the spiritual, moral, and religious education of the pahlavānān, this is the highest-ranking member within the zurxāne who plays the drum and bell while chanting poetry during exercises.

Narmeš: Stretches for mobility of the upper body.

Nowruz: The spring equinox festival.

Pā zadan ("Footwork"): Aerobic conditioning for nimbleness, speed, and dexterity.

Pahlavān ("Hero" or "Champion"): The morally and physically superior athlete of the zurxāne.

Rostam: The main hero of Iranian epic.

Sang: Wooden shields which are pressed upwards while prone on the ground. The purpose is to build excellent pushing and pressing strength, while in a state of motion, rather than in a static position used in the modern bench press.

Sharī'a: Islamic law.

Shī'a: A predominantly Persian branch of Islam that considers the Prophet Muḥammad's son-in-law 'Alī ibn Abī Ṭāleb to be his successor. The Shī'ītes take their name from Shī'at 'Alī, meaning "Partisans of 'Alī."

Ṣufīsm: An esoteric Muslim sect strongly influenced by Iranian Buddhism, which aims at the overcoming of the lower self through spiritual development.

Taxte-ye šeno: Push-up boards.

Vara: An underground shelter to protect humans from the coming Malkosan ("Evil Winters"), built by Yima and filled with waters and grassland.

Varzeš-e Pahlavāni: The Persian tradition of training in physical practices geared towards fighting, using tools that emulate weapons of war.

Vay: The wind god with both light and dark traits, associated with the warrior band in both Avestan and Vedic cultures.

Vərəthragna ("Obstruction Smiter"): The god of victory who slays enemies in battle and brings disease and death to those who deceive Mithra. He epitomises the ideal of an "Aryan warrior."

Vourukaša: The Cosmic Ocean upon which the earth floats as a disc.

Xamgiri: Leg stretches and squats done in preparation for swinging the mil, and as a way of recovering after the šeno exercises.

Xvarənah: The pure, all-luminous substance of which all of Ohrmazd's creatures are constituted at their origin. He is the Energy of sacral Light ensuring victory for the Forces of Light over the demonic Powers of Darkness. Not an abstract concept, but a real, physical, though invisible force – the creative power of the gods.

Yasna ("Sacrifice"): Particularly to the fire, this practice was central to pre-Islamic Iranian religion.

Yasna Hapanghaīti: A part of the Avesta.

Zand: A commentary on the ancient and incomprehensible prayers and hymns of Zoroastrianism.

Zarathuštra: The prophet to whom the Gāthās are attributed, and on whose teachings Zoroastrianism is based.

Zoroastrianism: A somewhat syncretic pre-Islamic Iranian religion based on the teachings of the prophet Zarathuštra and subsequent Avestan writings, and the worship of Ahura Mazdā (Ohrmazd). This was the first notably dualistic religion, inspiring the later Abrahamic iterations thereof.

Zurxāne: A place where warriors, heroes, and athletes train. It is a sacred space that has had a home in the Indo-European warrior soul since time immortal.

WarYoga Zurxāne

Was written by Tom Billinge.

Learn more about WarYoga at **WarYoga.com**, and Tom Billinge at **TomBillinge.com**.

If you enjoyed this book, consider reading *WarYoga* and the *Heroes of Greek Myth* series, also by Tom Billinge.

Watch for future releases by Tom and other authors from Sanctus Arya Press.

EX UMBRA IN SOLEM

www.ingramcontent.com/pod-product-compliance
Lightning Source LLC
Chambersburg PA
CBHW082035230426
43670CB00016B/2664